PLANT-POWERED
MEN

PLANT-POWERED
MEN

Inspirational Men Share their Secrets of
Optimal Health and Boundless Energy

Compiled by
Kathy Divine

Plant-powered Men is a series of papers submitted by, and interviews conducted with, vegan men from around the world.

The author and contributors to this publication shall not be liable in any action, claims or proceedings arising out of any information provided in this publication, nor shall they be responsible for any errors or omissions in such information. They expressly disclaim all and any liability to any person or persons arising out of anything done, or omitted to be done, in association with the publication of this book. The publication does not purport to provide medical advice or opinion and readers should not rely upon any information which is contained in this publication for that purpose. Any reader wishing to obtain medical advice or opinion should consult his or her own health professional.

Please consult the appropriate well-informed health professional if you are contemplating making a lifestyle or dietary change.

Editor: Julie Dixon
Cover design: Shuang Wu
Vegans Are Cool logo: Sam Shen: www.beveg.cn

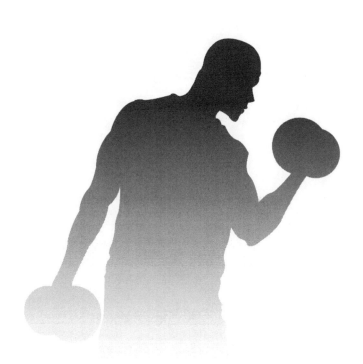

Dedicated to men everywhere
seeking healthier, happier lives.

ACKNOWLEDGMENTS

A HUGE THANK YOU to the plant-powered men who contributed their time, energy and passion to this project. By sharing your knowledge, experience and thoughts about your plant-powered lifestyle, you have brought this project to life.

Julie Dixon, the editor of *Plant-powered Men*, is the perfect combination of technical skill, creativity and intelligence. Without Julie this book would not have happened. I'm sure of it. Her input cannot be underestimated and I will be forever grateful for her contribution. My very humble thanks to you Julie!

Shuang Wu, thank you for your creativity, design expertise, ongoing enthusiasm and all-round commitment to the project. You are amazing!

A huge thank you to Richard Watts for his input on the cover design. Your support and assistance is much appreciated. Likewise to Amanda Benham, Tara Lomax and Sy Woon for their advice and fact-checking assistance. Not forgetting Mark Berriman for the use of his extensive vegan library to assist with background research and for his editing assistance.

Last but certainly not least, a huge thank you to my Facebook friends and fans of the Vegans Are Cool Facebook page for your feedback and ideas. My sincere thanks to you all.

CONTENTS

INTRODUCTION

WHY IS IT that humans think a meat-based, or omnivorous, diet is the key to energy and strength? There are an increasing number of people taking the lead from the elephants and their plant-eating pals by adopting a plant-powered diet. They are finding that their energy is skyrocketing, their strength and endurance increasing and their overall health improving tremendously.

They also feel happy and secure in the knowledge that they are avoiding a huge list of lifestyle diseases such as heart disease, colon cancer and type-two diabetes, to name just a few.

Despite the evidence from the animal kingdom that a plant-based diet is the diet of giants and strong guys (just look at the gorillas and giraffes), men have been raised to believe that eating animal products is essential for a strong, healthy body – that it is superior to plant-based eating. Through my interviews with men for my blog www.vegansarecool.com and interviews for my previous two books *Forever 21* and *Vegans Are Cool,* I had the opportunity to meet and read incredible stories about healthy, strong men – many of them athletes –

who are discovering that their plant-powered (vegan) diet is giving them an advantage in many aspects of their lives. Vegan men are a true inspiration to me and I am absolutely thrilled to be able to share their stories, tips and advice with you.

When compiling this book I strived for diversity – in age, occupation, personality and culture. There is representation from all inhabited continents (apart from Antarctica!) with men ranging in age from 22 to 71, including doctors, artists, teachers and scientists. My aim was to illustrate that plant-powered men are everywhere and come from all walks of life.

There were some common themes that emerged from the contributors – most frequent being the energy and vitality that the plant-powered diet has given them. Enhanced health, physical endurance and stamina were common benefits cited. A number of men talked about the emergence of their compassion for animals; I found this to be particularly revealing. I was really touched to read all of these very open and honest accounts. There is also a lot of humour (with one submission from a vegan comedian!).

A few notes regarding style: we have maintained American English for American submissions, and British English for British submissions and so on. Apart from these differences, we have attempted to maintain a consistent style throughout the book while allowing each writer to express his individuality and creativity.

All submissions were in written form, some choosing to submit essays while others preferred to do a "Q & A" style.

Every contributor to this book is committed to eating a plant-powered diet – they eat exclusively from the plant kingdom and do not eat any animal products including red meat, chicken, fish, dairy products and eggs or anything else that comes from an animal. They are also all vegan. This means that they avoid the use of animal products in all aspects of their lives (such as the use of leather and wool, as well as personal hygiene and household products). I encourage you to check out the photos of these amazing men at www. vegansarecool.com/men.

I really enjoyed connecting with the 38 men who wrote for the book and I know you'll enjoy connecting with them, too, as you join them on their plant-powered journey.

Plant-powered Men clearly illustrates that many men are benefiting immensely from a vegan diet. I sincerely hope that you will also be inspired to live a healthier life.

Kathy Divine

1

The Athletes, Powerlifters and Fitness-focused Men

A NEW BREED OF man is helping to redefine notions of masculinity. Ideas of integrity, compassion, kindness, moral strength, alignment to ethical values as well as traditional notions of physical might and courage are shaping a new paradigm of what it means to be a man in this century. In this chapter we'll meet ten very inspiring men who embody this new ideal of masculinity. They hail from different walks of life, nationalities and age groups yet have two things in common: all have excelled in their chosen sport or physical pursuit and all have done so while adhering to a plant-based diet. In this chapter we'll follow their personal journeys, learn about the books and DVDs that influenced them and hear their secrets to "bullet-proof" health, age-defying physical strength and fitness and "fountain-of-youth" appeal and vitality.

Being a Vegan Man[1]

David Rafter
Australia

Growing up as the youngest of ten children, I assure you there were more than a few initiations into the ranks of being a man – you don't have five brothers without getting knocked around a bit. Although I never played physical-contact sports such as rugby union, rugby league or AFL, my parents made sure we played pretty much every other sport under the sun: swimming, baseball, athletics, surfing, and of course tennis. Looking back on it, I guarantee my parents were just trying to tire us out so we would go to bed at night.

I find that living in a culture such as Australia's, it is almost expected of a man that he play lots of sport and love his barbecue – and I shouldn't just say Australia: if you look at most Western cultures, it's very much like this. In my family, it was no different; in fact, if anything, that culture was more intense when our brother Pat started to perform very well on the tennis tour. When someone close to you starts to do very well in his or her chosen sport, it seems your life revolves around them; their wins become your wins, and their losses become your losses. I remember watching the Wimbledon final in 2001: it was purely devastating watching our beautiful brother lose in the final. You knew how much he wanted it, and you could feel some

---

1   A version of this article originally appeared in *Vegans Are Cool* (2011).

of the pain he must have been going through. It really is as if your whole family becomes one.

So, you could only imagine that when Patty started to focus on his dietary intake to improve his physical condition, the whole family became involved. It is a wonderful feeling having so many people connected in your life, but at the same time it can be hard to break the mould. When you speak to some of the "old school" doctors, they are very much inundated with the dogma of the traditional medical system: you need to have meat to get your iron, and milk to get your calcium and eggs...well, they make you fart to get rid of all the other stuff in your system, I joke.

You remember that food pyramid that outlines where you get all your dietary vitamins and minerals? When I look at it now, it seems so outdated and fatigued. It almost looks like a chart that the old doctors drew up in the 1950s about how smoking is good for you so that tobacco companies could increase their sales.

As I mentioned earlier, I had always been a very physical person. I love getting out on my surfboard and catching a few waves, or going for a run in the national park. To me, it is an amazing relief. It is like all the stresses from the world just go, and you are at one with yourself and the world. However, as you could imagine, the moment that I told my family I was vegan, all these questions and statements popped out of nowhere: "David, how are you going to get your iron?," "David how are you going to get vitamin B12, you know your

body needs it!," "David you are too skinny." Those
of you out there who have made the transition to the
vegan diet, might have already heard some of these.
They don't seem to happen once or twice either: you
seem to get bombarded with them (although I can
assure you they do stop).

I can still remember the time I made the choice to drop
animal products from my diet. I was doing my normal
run through the Noosa National Park which went for
30 minutes. When I was coming to the end, I could feel
I could keep on going – I just kept up the pace, and
an hour went by and my body still felt amazing. I felt
I could keep on running and running. I was picturing
myself being Forrest Gump running across Australia
– I can assure you I had the beard to match. It was a
remarkable experience to feel your body feel so light
you could really run the whole day – and it was more
remarkable to think that by simply making the choice to
drop meat and dairy from my diet, it would have such
an impact on the condition of my body.

I can also recall a time I was surfing with a couple of
my brothers. We had been out for most of the day,
having a ball, catching some great waves. I paddled into
one wave, pushed myself up to stand up on the board,
and I thought I could literally fly. I felt so light and agile
I really did think I was going to take off and go for a
little trip – such a breathtaking experience.

To be honest with you, however, the constant remarks
I was getting from my family and friends were getting

to me. I took the time to get regular iron and vitamin B12 tests. The whole time, throughout all my physical activities and dietary changes, no doctors could find anything abnormal in my blood. In fact, I went to give blood and the nurses could not believe how high my iron level was.

So, if you are a man living on this beautiful planet and you have made the choice to transition to the compassionate vegan lifestyle, and you still love your sport, here are a few tips that might be good for keeping your dietary needs in check:

» Do eat your greens, and if you can, get into green smoothies. Eating green leafy vegetables is a great way to get iron, especially if you can eat them raw. When you eat the vegetable in its natural state, you harness all of its nutritional value.

» Do your best to stay away from heavy foods such as chocolate, chips, bread and pasta. They can have an adverse effect on your body and in fact cause depletion of other minerals and vitamins.

» Instead, look to grains such as quinoa, brown rice, and even millet. Not only are they filling and the carbohydrate your body could be looking for, they have a high level of protein and are full of all the amino acids.

» Another great source for you to get your protein from is legumes such as lentils, soy beans and peas such as chickpeas. To be honest, though, I don't eat a lot of soy, but I do really enjoy a beautiful dahl (a lentil dish).

» Get stuck into your fruit, especially bananas and berries such as strawberries and blueberries. They are high in fibre and chock-full of magnesium and potassium to give you that energy boost.

When I was initially making the transition to the vegan diet, I really watched the amount of heavy foods I was having, because I knew that foods such as bread, pasta, chocolate and chips cause your body to slow down. You will really notice this effect when you put these foods into your system. According to the evidence, the nutritional value of foods such as breads, pasta and grains provides your body with a high level of carbohydrates. Personally, I have never felt I needed that carbohydrate in my system in order to perform physical activity. I have never noticed my body getting tired; in fact, as I mentioned earlier, I felt I had a lot more energy. Though, on another note, please do listen to your body. If you are doing a lot of activity and you are feeling tired, look at increasing your carbohydrates and make sure you are eating enough legumes and greens so you're getting your iron.

Don't be too alarmed if when you first go vegan, you receive some of the remarks I mentioned earlier. Your loved ones are just concerned for you, and they love you very much. Keep in mind they have been raised on the "old school" food pyramid, and that their "old school" doctors might not know any different.

If you're finding that it's tough, make sure you surround yourself with like-minded people. Find yourself a good doctor who has done his or her research and who is in line with your new found lifestyle. Just because you're a man and have become vegan doesn't mean you have to drop all the things you used to love to do. You can sit down with your family and friends and enjoy the Friday-night game or go out for a surf. Anyway, your friends might even be jealous of you because your whole being is radiating now, and all the girls are flocking to you.

Connect with David:

www.veganera.com
www.facebook.com/VeganEra

Plant-powered Body Building

Richard Watts
UK

I have been vegan since the end of 2000, so at the time of writing, I have been vegan for about 12 years. Before that I was vegetarian for about 13 years. Unfortunately, most people who read that would assume I am skin and bone, and it is a miracle I haven't died from malnutrition yet. Actually, I am in fine health, and often have people remark on my physical condition. Indeed, I've inspired many people to get back to the gym –

whether they know I'm vegan or not, they ask me what I've been doing to get in shape – so I feel proud that I'm a positive example of a vegan. I work as a labourer at an animal sanctuary, which is a pretty physical job. Also on my days off I go to the gym for weight training. I run the website veganbodybuilding.com, and I was asked to write this article to give some insight into training, diet and health on a vegan diet. But I think I should rewind and start with some fundamentals.

It seems that vegetarianism is far easier for most people to understand, than veganism. The idea that for meat to exist, an animal had to die is easy to comprehend. Veganism is often considered to be going "too far" or "unnecessary", or even just completely pointless. However, there are two key facts that really need to be appreciated.

First, in order to get a cow to produce milk, she needs to be impregnated, just like a human. Male calves born in this process obviously do not produce milk themselves. Thinking about this from a business perspective, there is nothing to gain by having billions of male calves on your land, serving no purpose. The only thing they can do is provide semen for breeding (for which you only need a tiny number of males). With that being the case, most are killed for meat. So in order to get milk from dairy cows, there is this side effect of the male calves having to be killed, that's a fact.

Similarly with eggs, you need female chickens to lay more eggs. Male chickens serve no purpose and represent no profit to the farmer, so the general system is to kill them, normally immediately when the chicks are identified as male. Obviously a few males are required for breeding, so a few might live. But if you buy eggs, then part of the process of how you get the egg, involves the slaughter of billions of male chickens, there's no other way around it.

With that said, the question of "what's wrong with milk and eggs" becomes very simple – there is a lot more to be said, but the bottom line is that in order to produce milk or eggs, there are billions of males being killed constantly. As a person who cares about animals, it is the same choice as a vegetarian choosing not to eat meat.

But it is strange to me that often it is considered not to be masculine if you show compassion, caring, or even kindness – and that lack of masculinity is magnified if those feelings are towards animals. I think that's absolutely nuts. It's just sensible to not want harm to come to anything. Given a choice between something being harmed, or not being harmed, why would you want to choose the first option? It's often misconstrued as weak, or overly emotional, but it's just logical, just straight forward. To actually want something to be harmed is sadistic.

But I think the lack of consideration towards animals is generally limited to men. Women I have talked to are usually impressed by veganism, even if they are not vegan or even vegetarian themselves, they can see that I am someone who takes himself seriously, has self-respect, pride and whose word means something. If you make a commitment to something like veganism, it shows a dedication and belief in something beyond your own life. It's easy to just say the words, "I care about animals" and so on. Unless you actually change your lifestyle, it's basically nonsense – how can you say you care about something, when you pay for someone to kill it so you can eat it? When faced with someone who follows through with their actions, it shows that they believe in what they say and their words carry much more weight. Of course, there is also the other side of it; that women perhaps find it more comfortable to feel empathy in general, and so it is refreshing for them to meet a man who is unafraid to also show compassion towards animals.

But once you accept that killing animals is wrong, the world takes on a very different appearance. It infuriates me, and the emotion I feel most is anger. I take it for granted that cruelty and slaughter of animals is wrong now – I have been vegan for so long it's not something I think about. Veganism is not some kind of hippy, fluffy nonsense. To me it's more about being so enraged with what's going on, that you put your foot down and say "no". It takes some guts to do something different, to stand out and let your beliefs dictate your actions. It's easy – and weak – to just go with the flow, join in with your friends, not make a fuss. I think it underlies real strength to be true to yourself and what you consider to be right, or wrong. It seems repulsive to me that in order to be considered to be a "real man", you have to take pleasure in the suffering of animals. That seems so backwards.

I also despise the notion of masculinity in general. To define men as one thing and women as another is just discrimination. Who makes the rules? Why are certain sports "for men" and others "for women"? It is completely fabricated. Sure, there are trends regarding how men and women behave and interact, and even how they think. But those are only trends, not rules. There is no reason to consider any action or activity as "male" or "female". My interests are varied, and include things that some might call masculine, and others feminine. I like to lift weights, practice martial arts, listen to heavy metal and play guitar, play video games, read graphic novels, watch action movies and horror, and have an interest in serial killers. Then, I also like Bob Ross, origami, drawing and painting, playing with kittens, cooking, watching dramas and documentaries, and I have no problem talking to people about their feelings and what is going on in their life.

To me, it's all the same. Neither list has a gender associated with it. And what does it say about me if you did arbitrarily associate a gender? I don't like being pigeonholed, I'm an individual like everybody else, with interests, likes and dislikes. Anybody can do anything they like, and there should not be a stigma attached to it. Caring about animals is a logical practice, not something which should be looked down upon as childish or "girly".

But even for those who understand, or even agree, that animal farming is unacceptable, there are further issues to do with the application and practicality of veganism that need addressing. These are some common questions I get asked, and I'll do my best to explain.

Where do you get your protein?

A big concern for people about veganism is protein. But, I don't think many people even know how much protein you're supposed to get in a day, they just assume they get enough if they eat meat, and assume you don't get enough if you are vegan or vegetarian. However, if you look at information from official health guidelines around the world, including the World Health Organisation, the recommendations for everyday average people is that between five to ten per cent of your calories should come from protein.

Protein is easy to come by on a vegan diet. Protein is everywhere, not limited to animal products! Just for example:

Spinach – 32% calories from protein
Kidney beans – 24% calories from protein
Bread – 12% calories from protein
Rice – 8% calories from protein
Oats – 12 % calories from protein
Peanuts – 15% calories from protein
Cashews – 11% calories from protein
Green Peas – 22% calories from protein

(numbers taken from nutritiondata.com)

So you can see, that even with just regular fresh foods and staples, you would easily reach that recommendation of five to ten percent. Those are just examples, but if you have a look around at the nutritional data of foods, you might be surprised how easy it is to get it in your diet. In fact, I believe it is harder to avoid it than it is to obtain it. If you eat enough calories in a day, your diet would have to be really peculiar to completely miss the mark. Basically the only people who don't get enough protein, are those who are starving in general, who don't get enough calories.

Can you build muscle as a vegan?

Yeah. If you find the time, you can check veganbodybuilding.com and you can see in the profiles section, dozens of examples of fit and healthy people, as well as some really huge and ripped guys. Building muscle as a vegan is the same process as building muscle as a non-vegan. Primarily, you need to train hard and consistently towards a set goal, and eat appropriately. Everyone has a different goal in mind, but generally I guess most everyday people want to get a bit bigger, and get a bit leaner. At a simplistic level, that means eating enough carbohydrates to allow you to function properly and exercise, and eating enough protein to help you recover after your workouts.

There is continuing disagreement and discussion about how much protein somebody should consume if they are trying to put on muscle. Some people talk about having one gram of protein for every pound of bodyweight. So if you weigh 150 pounds, some would say you should consume 150 grams of protein every day. Others even say double that amount! Personally I've seen progress from people eating far less than that. But really it involves personal experimentation. Create a diet plan, stick to it for three months or so, see if you get the changes you want, and then go from there, making alterations. There isn't a magic recipe that will turn you into the hulk, no matter if you're vegan, vegetarian or a meat-eater. It requires dedication and hard work, that's the key. Often, bodybuilders consume protein shakes as a convenient way to get additional protein in their diet, with minimum additional calories. Again, that is true of vegans, vegetarians and meat-eaters (the latter often consume whey, whilst vegans would be on something like soy or rice protein and so on).

Don't vegans miss something in their diet? Isn't it unhealthy?

It depends on the diet. Somebody who eats meat is not intrinsically healthier than someone who doesn't, and vice versa. I know some very unhealthy people, and I know some extremely healthy people. I'd say that anybody hoping to be healthy needs to make sure they're eating a high quantity of fruits and vegetables. That should be the bulk of your diet, no matter what else you're consuming. So even if somebody doesn't want to be vegetarian or vegan, I'd say that they should still focus on fruit and vegetables just for their health, if nothing else. I would also say that the more animal products you consume, the worse it will be for your health, especially those that are known to contribute to cancer and heart disease. Exclusion of animal products does nothing to harm you. Veganism is certainly not dangerous to your health. It's impossible to say "you'll be healthier if you become vegan" – because you might become vegan and then just start eating chips and candy. Obviously that is not healthy at all, but that would be your own ignorance causing the health problems, not veganism. The only thing I would say you need to remember as a vegan, is to make sure you are eating foods fortified with vitamin B12, or take a supplement for that vitamin, as it will only be in fortified foods (like cereal), and if you're not eating those, then you likely won't be getting much of it.

There is a lot more to cover than I have in this brief article, and I'm sure that other contributors to this book will have their own perspectives and advice. But I think that nobody should shy away from veganism on the grounds that it is "feminine", unfashionable or unhealthy. I really recommend doing your homework before reaching any conclusion. Make a diet plan, look at what you currently eat, check out nutritiondata.com or a similar site to understand precisely how much fat, carbohydrate and protein you eat per day, and how many calories you take in. It'll take you a little while, maybe an hour, depending on the complexity of your diet. But then you'll have the facts. I think most people do not know how much they eat – let alone what they should be eating! But once you start putting a diet together, and trying to optimize it, you can achieve a very healthy plan as a vegan.

Connect with Richard:

www.veganbodybuilding.com

Why Eating Fruits and Vegetables is Lifesaving

John Lewis
USA

Name: John Lewis
Age: 35
Occupation: health consultant, motivational speaker
and founder of Bad Ass Vegan
Vegan since: 2007
Best thing about being vegan: enlightening the
souls of the planet including animals and the human
race and in turn improving my health.

What prompted you to make the shift to a vegan diet? How is it working for you?

Well I was already vegetarian for quite a few years and
the extra research I did led me to become a vegan.
Another factor was the fact that my mother had
developed colon cancer and after doing my research
about how it was caused and actually talking to doctors,
it was revealed to me that too much animal protein and
fried foods and things of that nature helped this disease
develop within her system. Being a vegan is working
out wonderfully for me, there's no turning back now
especially with my health as great as it is.

What is your favourite vegan food?

That is a tricky question to answer. I love vegan food. If I had to pick one dish it most likely would be my dish I call "a beautiful mess". The dish consists of steamed quinoa, raw spinach, one Hass avocado, which becomes a guacamole style sauce. Mix it all together and you have a beautiful mess.

What are the benefits of being vegan for you?

There are many benefits to being a vegan but the major benefit for me is being an athlete and being able to train extra hard and having a speedy recovery time to train just as hard the next day. It's also a great benefit just to be able to know that along with my training, if I eat plant-based fuel I will be able to avoid many diseases that plague so many individuals.

What advice would you give men who are considering the switch to the vegan lifestyle?

First bit of advice: avoid negativity. You will run into a lot of people that will second guess your decision. One of my favorite things to say to people is that if you go and look at any hospital and check all the rooms in the hospital you will come to one conclusion: the hospital is not full of people that eat fruits and vegetables.

Do you feel strong and healthy as a vegan man?

Not only do I feel stronger but more importantly I feel connected to my body. I'm able to understand that the nutrients from the food are helping me and that when

I workout with purpose each muscle gains with each workout. So in short yes, I feel strong and this is only the beginning.

Connect with John:

www.badassvegan.com

The Many Benefits of Plant-powered Living

Dan Schulz
Australia

Name: Dan Schulz
Age: 38
Occupation: marketing consultant to the wellness industry
Vegan since: 1994
Best thing about being vegan: peace of mind

What prompted you to make the shift to a vegan diet?

I was always fascinated with the human body and the fact that you could improve it and repair it by simply choosing the right food and exercise while avoiding anything toxic. While studying anatomy and physiology at university I dissected human bodies along with the bodies of various animals, comparing their digestive systems and studying research into effects of different diets on humans; even volunteering myself as a subject for experiments related to nutrition and muscle performance.

While doing my Masters degree I became the first undergraduate student to have his research published in an international medical journal.

My studies convinced me that the human body was intelligently designed and designed to eat plant foods only.

Throughout my youth I lifted weights in my spare time and desired to be big and strong. The recommendation from all the fitness magazines I was reading was that a high protein diet was essential for building muscle and that the *only* way to get a lot of protein was eating animals. Despite what I was learning at university about the health benefits of a plant-based diet the idea of being healthy yet thin and scrawny prevented me from becoming vegan.

Then I read *Fit For Life* by Harvey Diamond. There was a section in the book that talked about silverback gorillas being strong enough to pick up a man with one hand and throw him around like a frisbee and that they only ate fruit and leaves. That mental imagery had a powerful effect on me. Nothing could be more macho than being as strong as a gorilla, right?

When I finished reading the last page I became 100 per cent vegan. My concerned grandparents went to see their doctor and told him that their grandson had decided to become vegan. The doctor told them that I would die if I did not eat meat. Nineteen years later and I'm not only still alive, I'm strong enough to pick that doctor up and throw him around like a frisbee.

The week after reading *Fit For Life* I started a massage course. I was going to university, massage college and working a night job all at the same time. I did not have time to eat more than the odd bit of fruit so for three weeks I was on a fruit fast while being massaged five days a week.

As a result my 120 kilogram (264 pound) body shed 30 kilograms (66 pounds) within that three week period; the whole time having flu-like symptoms yet actually feeling good. I was going to the toilet almost hourly and blowing my nose constantly.

How is it working for you?

It has been life changing in only good ways, no negatives.

After massage school, I started eating normal amounts of food and my body quickly rebuilt itself. Prior to becoming vegan I was frequently sick, particularly with head colds. I spent the first 19 years of my life blowing my nose daily. In the 19 vegan years that followed I have never been sick. The exceptions have been only twice in 19 years where I got a head cold but on both occasions it took extreme exhaustion, dehydration, sleep deprivation and hypothermia to put me out of action for 24 hours. Unless I experience all four of those things simultaneously my health remains bullet-proof.

I also learned how to attain and maintain high amounts of vitamin B12 without supplements, without fortified foods, no synthetics, just eating plants. A common criticism of a vegan diet is that this is not possible.

A well-known naturopath heard this about me so invited me to come in for blood and urine tests to see if it was true. I had the first perfect blood and urine tests she had seen. I then got invited to talk about it on television. The producers of the television program edited out the part where I reveal the secret so you'll have to contact me if you want to learn what it is.

Something else that happened shortly after switching to being vegan was that my aggressive tendencies subsided and I developed a real love and respect for animals, something I previously did not have.

So in addition to changing my diet for health reasons I also changed other areas of my life to remove any and all objects made from animals. It is not difficult to find beautiful clothes, shoes, deodorants, skin and hair products, furniture etc. that are made without animals.

I also adopted some dogs that were raised as meat eaters and switched them to vegan diets with the addition of some medicinal foods like hemp and mangosteen. The (very rapid) changes I noticed were improved mood, shinier coats, cessation of arthritis, cessation of bad breath and no further need of pain and seizure medication. They are really happy, healthy dogs.

What is your favourite vegan food?

That's easy - hemp foods! I eat a *lot* of hemp seeds and hemp protein powder and have never felt better and been stronger. Hemp turns scrawn into brawn. If you could see my strength gains on a graph you'd see they closely follow how much hemp I eat. The more hemp I eat the younger I look and feel.

Here's a smoothie I have daily:

- » 6 tablespoons of hemp protein powder
- » 2 tablespoons of hemp seeds
- » 1 banana
- » half a cup of blueberries
- » 1 teaspoon of cinnamon
- » a few drops of stevia
- » 2 cups of filtered cold water

This is a great muscle-building smoothie that keeps blood sugar low, allows growth hormone to stay high after exercise and during sleep, floods your body with enough branched chain amino acids to have an anabolic effect on your metabolism and helps reduce inflammation by supplying all the essential fatty acids you need. You'll recover quicker and get stronger.

What are the benefits of being vegan for you?

There are plenty. I enjoy eating delicious meals that actually clean my body rather than clog it and I feel strong and healthy all the time. I also enjoy having a clean conscience. The fountain of youth is found in plant foods.

It was particularly interesting to read the Bible later in life and discover that according to the Bible God designed humans to eat plant foods. The first two and last two pages of the Bible contain instructions on what to eat in order to achieve optimum health and how to reverse disease.

Once you make a concerted effort to only give your body clean water and clean foods that are made from fruits, vegetables, seeds and greens your mind and body keep improving. It's the only thing that works 100 per cent of the time for 100 per cent of people.

What advice would you give men who are considering the switch to the vegan lifestyle?

Eat hemp.
Eat hemp.

Go exploring your local whole foods markets and restaurants and find vegan foods that you enjoy the taste of. Your taste buds will likely have more decision-making power than your brain does. Convince yourself that the pleasure of eating will still be there and the rest is easy.

In Australia there are a few standout places where you can find such food. Iku in Sydney and Shakahari and Vegebar in Melbourne are my favorite places to get delicious vegan meals. I get hemp foods from Hemp Foods Australia www.hempfoods.com.au and use body products from Pure & Green Organics www.pureandgreen.com.au.

Do you feel strong and healthy as a vegan man?

I'm 6'7" and can lift trees – I'm much stronger and much healthier than in my non-vegan days.

Anything else you would like to add?

Guys – impotence, bad breath, bad skin, heart disease, arthritis, flatulence, obesity and animal torture are not sexy or macho. If for no other reason than being more attractive, start discovering delicious plant-based foods. The 2012 movie *Forks Over Knives* (www.forksoverknives. com) does a pretty good job of covering the facts; it's inspiring and enlightening, enjoyable and easy to watch. In Australia you can buy it from www.myflix.com.au

Other than that, expect but ignore critics and know that there are powerful, well-funded organizations that desperately do not want you to have this information. They want you to believe that eating animals is safe and will make you popular while being vegan is risky and fanatical. They do this by influencing media, entertainment, education and government and succeed in deceiving many respected health "authorities" that black is white and bad is good.

Don't be fooled. Prove it to yourself. Real men are healthy, strong, youthful and compassionate and they make up their own minds so don't let some obese, smelly, impotent arthritic PR executive tell you what to do with your body.

Connect with Dan:

I'm happy to answer "how to" questions about food, strength and other aspects of a vegan lifestyle: dan@ edan.com.au.

Getting the Edge, Vegan Style

Brandden Lassells
USA/Australia

Name: Brandden Lassells
Age: 71
Occupation: harp maker
Vegan since: vegetarian and/or vegan since the 1970s, and a period as vegan from 1986 to 1996, then vegetarian only and now, since 2007, 100 per cent committed vegan.
Best thing about being vegan: the energy and good health it brings plus the good vibes from having compassion for animals and the planet.

What prompted you to make the shift to a vegan diet? How is it going?

Finally woke up in 2007, realised that the best I felt was when I was vegan earlier in my life and also read some information on veganism which enlightened me and made me totally aware of why being vegan is the only sensible way to live.

What is your favourite vegan food?

Organic raw fruit, organic raw veggie salads as well as organic steamed brown rice.

What are the benefits of being vegan for you?

Increased energy and wellbeing as well as feeling good about doing my part for the animals and the planet.

What advice would you give men who are considering the switch to the vegan lifestyle?

Once you educate yourself about all of the benefits and reasons for leading a vegan lifestyle there can be little choice but that the vegan lifestyle is the way we are meant to live. Get past all the myths about protein and especially the need for dairy. Once you decide to follow a vegan path I recommend only being in a relationship with another vegan so that you can share values. In my case, although admittedly a weakness on my part, I was vegan many years ago and then after being in a relationship with a vegetarian, I found it difficult to remain vegan with the dietary differences. Once you become aware of the virtues of being vegan it will not make sense to compromise your diet and kitchen. It will be a joy to share this lifestyle with someone with the same values.

Do you feel strong and healthy as a vegan man?

Most definitely and I feel younger than my chronological age too. I would like to add that in the late 80s and early 90s during the time I was completely vegan I was also a highly successful oarsman competing in world championships and also rowing in what is called open water rowing (rowing long distance across open ocean or other water). During this time I was in my mid 40s and early 50s. In the open water rowing which is akin to running a marathon, I won just about every race I entered and set many records – all the while competing against men much my junior and even Olympians. In the Masters sprint rowing I often competed against younger aged men as well as those of my own age and I was a very consistent winner and never went to a local or World Masters Rowing championship without taking at least two gold medals. All the while other competitors could not fathom how this older man who only consumed a plant-based diet could be so healthy and successful. When interviewed the topic of my diet was usually raised with disbelief – but the proof of the virtues of being vegan is in the results.

Anything else you would like to add?

Any truly thinking and educated man would not be anything but vegan.

Fitness Tips from a Plant-powered Physiotherapist

Ryan McKeough
Canada

Name: Ryan McKeough BKiH, MPhysio
Occupation: physiotherapist
Age: 25
Vegan since: 2011
Best thing about being vegan: always having the energy to train hard. Staying lean and toned without needing to calorie count or do lots of cardio. And knowing I'm making a difference in changing how the world views non-human animals.

What inspired you to go vegan?

I was the typical meat and potatoes kind of guy and just happened to stumble upon the *Meet Your Meat* video. I couldn't sleep that night. I had always considered myself an animal lover, and after seeing what has to happen for meat to arrive on my plate, I realised that I could not continue to support such an industry and decided to go vegetarian.

It was a few years later when I finally got the kick I needed to go vegan. I had been looking more into the cruel practices of the dairy and egg industry and was pretty convinced that it wasn't something I could support, but what finally made me make the switch was an incident in the classroom whilst studying for my Masters degree.

A classmate of mine had told me she was considering going from vegetarian to vegan, and many of the men in the class began to really grill her about it (no pun intended), telling her about how bad it was for her health. I spoke up and said that it was a perfectly healthy diet, but I realised that if I actually made the switch myself, I would be speaking much louder with my actions. So I decided that to support her I myself would make the transition, and I've never looked back. She hasn't made the switch yet, but I have faith in her!

Is the vegan diet good for health in your opinion?

Definitely! I'm someone who really weighs logic and fact when making a decision. I wouldn't be vegan if it weren't shown to be a perfectly healthy diet with scientific research and organisations supporting that fact. Look no further than the American Dietetic Association's (the largest dietetic body in the world) official stance on the vegan diet to see the answer.

You look really strong and fit! What do you eat to maintain a good fitness level?

I follow a pretty typical vegan diet filled with whole grains, beans (including soy products), lentils and legumes, nuts, seeds and a large variety of fruit and vegetables. It's what I don't put into my body that helps me stay lean and fit. I shun greasy foods like chips, and pass on sweets such as cakes and lollies. What really makes the difference however, is exercise. Diet is only half of the battle!

Do you have a typical daily menu? If so, what do you eat?

I'll tend to do a workout in the morning before work, and follow it with a protein shake and something like a peanut butter sandwich and a banana. I'll snack on almonds, fruit, or sticks of vegetables throughout the morning if I have the time, and have what's left over from dinner the night before for lunch. That's usually some form of stir fry with a healthy grain like quinoa or couscous with vegetables and a protein source like tofu, lentils, kidney beans, etc. Dinner is usually a similarly styled meal, consisting of a grain, several veggies, and a protein source. I like to keep my meals pretty simple, call me a creature of habit!

Can men be fit and strong on a vegan diet?

Absolutely. The idea that animal protein is necessary to be strong and athletic is out-dated and pretty foolish. Look no further than the competitor profiles on www. veganbodybuilding.com to see that this concept is a myth. Carl Lewis, who many argue is the greatest track and fielder of all time, ran his best races on a vegan diet.

Making the switch will not harm your athletic performance or hinder your strength or fitness. I've achieved multiple personal bests for exercises in the gym while on a vegan diet, including a major goal of mine of bench-pressing 140 kilograms while at an 81 kilogram body weight. If you eat right and train hard, you get results. Eating vegan has the first part covered, the training part is up to you!

Do you have any fitness tips you would like to share?

I think that the term "fitness" is somewhat misconstrued nowadays. Fitness is more than just how you look and how you perform in the gym. How is your blood pressure? Cholesterol? How are the stress levels in your life? How do you feel about yourself as a person?

Fitness is something that should be looked at holistically, and this is the real reason why I feel that a vegan lifestyle is such a fantastic pathway to fitness. I am so much more at peace with myself based on the choices I've made, and I know I'm doing my heart a favour by eliminating cholesterol and nasty fats from my diet.

Some tips for exercise though? If you plan on starting, find a friend to start with you. It's a lot harder to hit the snooze button if you know you'll be letting your mate down. If you're uncertain about where to start, ask somebody! Any credible gym will have supervisors who should be glad to help you with any questions you have and may even design a program to help you reach your goals.

If you've been exercising for a while and seem to have plateaued with your gains, try to incorporate eccentric exercise into your routine. Eccentric exercise is the "down phase" of any exercise. So, imagine if you were doing a biceps curl, lowering the weight back down to your waist is the eccentric component. They are an excellent way to break through and achieve new personal bests.

Do you have any inspirational words for people thinking of switching to a vegan diet or starting a new fitness program?

Be proud of your decision to make a positive change in your life, as that is a truly significant step towards reaching your goal! Remember that everyone started from scratch at some point in his or her life, and that you have the potential to make any goal a reality if you're willing to put in the effort! Don't beat yourself up if you falter. Just remember that every time you take a step in the right direction, you're helping your mind lay the groundwork for making these new decisions part of your routine.

Any final words?

Vegans! We're making incredible progress in showing the world the benefits of this lifestyle, but we need to keep moving forward. To keep the ball rolling, every one of us needs to be the best person and ambassador that we can be for the vegan movement. That means showing strength in our convictions, keeping our minds and bodies healthy, and being open and honest about who and why we are who we are!

Gentlemen, if you're reading this then chances are either you or someone you care about is interested in you making the change. Be confident that you can do this, and be proud that you are making a great statement about who you are as an individual by living by a consistent moral code.

Yours in health, hope and happiness!

Achieving Optimal Health And Fitness

Jeff Sekerak
USA

Name: Jeff Sekerak
Age: 45
Occupation: real estate investor, author
Vegan since: 1992

Best thing about being vegan: superb health, from inside out as well as a greater connection with all beings (as you're not consuming them).

What prompted you to make the shift to a vegan diet? How is it working for you?

Originally, it was the reading of two books. First, Anthony Robbins', *Awaken The Giant Within*. And then, *Fit for Life* by Harvey Diamond. At the time I read these, over twenty years ago now, I was completely focused upon my sports performance. And Robbins, in his book, wrote briefly of the dangers of consuming animal protein, as well as the health benefits of consuming a more, plant-based fare. I did a bit of research on his work, and found it to be closely related, in overall philosophy, to Diamond's, *Fit for Life*.

So I read that as well. And that was it. After reading Harvey Diamond's break-down of the theory of natural hygiene, the horrific downside of consuming animal "foods", as well as the *great* benefits of consuming a largely, if not 100 per cent, plant-based diet, I became a vegan immediately. It's amazing how a single book can impact your life for the better. From that point on, I have not consumed animal products of any kind. How is it working? In a word, "beautifully".

Yes, I've had a few obstacles and hurdles along the way. If I had to do it all over again, I'd likely have gone with a more raw vegan approach, making fruits, from the start, rather than grains, the focus of my diet. Yet overall? Considering the shape I'm in physically, mentally, spiritually, after over two decades on a vegan diet? I couldn't be happier with it.

What is your favourite vegan food?

There are so many great ones, it's difficult to choose. I love mono-meals of mango. I love lemons, cucumber and spinach. Yet I suppose if I had to pick a single favorite dish, it would be this: a simple salad of squash, tomato, and spinach. The combination of non-sweet fruit, and mineral-rich greens, provides nearly every vitamin, mineral, amino acid, and essential fatty acid needed to sustain a healthy life. Also, it tastes great. Especially if you add a dash of sea salt, a bit of pepper and half a squeezed lemon upon it. And, perhaps most importantly, it fills you up as if you'd eaten a much heavier meal like one of rice, potatoes, etc. Yet the squash, tomato, and spinach salad, is *far* healthier, far easier to digest, and much lower in overall calories. You can't beat it.

What are the benefits of being vegan for you?

First, athletic performance. I've always played sports, and engaged in vigorous workouts. I played basketball and baseball in high school. Now my exercise regimen is one which would challenge a great number, I'm betting, of twenty-somethings. Yet I'm 45. So with the demanding exercise sessions I do daily, I've got to be aware of what I'm putting into my body, and its overall effect on my performance. An example? Well, just this morning, my workout was about 800 push-ups and crunches, along with an eight-mile run in home-made sandals. And I do that *at least* five days per week. Could I maintain that level of performance, eating burgers and fries? I doubt it.

Another benefit? Internal cleanliness. The vegan diet, rich in natural fiber, vitamins, and minerals, keeps the digestive tract cleansed, and is awash with *exactly* that which the body truly needs, in terms of nutrients. And the digestive system, this is where all disease begins. I'm in agreement with Professor Ehret (author of *The Mucusless Diet Healing System*), on that point. To be at your best, every cell in your body must be cleansed and free of obstructions. This *cannot* happen if you're consuming a high amount of fats, animal protein and dairy "foods", which only serve to clog the internal system beginning with the digestive tract, with indigestible, toxic material. That stuff builds up over time. Avoid it, and you'll be in great shape, throughout life, I've found. And you'll be fit for demanding workouts where others are not.

Another benefit? Mental clarity and sharpness. Again, it's pretty difficult to be at your best, in *any* way, when your internal "pipe system" is clogged with fats, animal proteins, and processed foods. These act as literal breeding grounds for unwanted, potentially harmful parasites. And the average person is loaded down with years worth of such toxins. In cases such as that? Well the digestive, and other systems, are so bogged down with unwanted material that the good things – the life-giving vitamins and minerals from raw plant-foods – cannot be digested properly, much less, assimilated.

This negatively impacts sleeping patterns, elimination patterns, and more. And when those issues arise, the mind *cannot* function at its best either. I've definitely noticed a far greater mental acuity, sharpness, even creativity since adopting the vegan diet. I'd never go back, to any other lifestyle. Not for any amount of money in the world.

Still another benefit? I've found you feel a whole lot better about yourself, spiritually-speaking, when you consume plants rather than other sentient beings. I consider all animals friends on our short journey on this planet. To eat some of them and simultaneously consider others as friends or pets is something I find to be totally incongruent, in philosophy. I think of it this way: most children, from a very early age, feel a deep connection, with animals, of all types. That connection forms a value system. Yet those values are compromised by learned behavior, as the child grows. He or she learns through commercial propaganda, and other sources, friends, family, etc., that eating animals is okay. Yet this is in direct contradiction with our natural, earliest-developed, true values. With this type of conflict going on inside one's soul it is - I know from personal experience, and from speaking with hundreds of others on the issue - nearly impossible to feel "grounded", spiritually-speaking.

So there you have, it. Just a few of the benefits of embracing the vegan lifestyle: physical, mental, spiritual. Again, I wouldn't change this, my chosen way of eating, for anything in the world.

What advice would you give men who are considering the switch to the vegan lifestyle?

Don't pay attention to the propaganda of the meat, dairy and processed-food industries: they are *more* than happy to delude you. They've been implying or directly stating, for generations, that without protein and dairy "foods", you might just wither away. You might end up with a calcium, or protein deficiency. And this, we know now, is completely inaccurate. We now know that humans, even avid athletes, require about six to ten per cent (and that ten per cent figure is high, I believe) of our calories from protein. That's about the amount contained in most fruits and vegetables. Most men are unaware of this. They're still under the impression that protein builds muscle. And in fact, there are no foods that do so. If you're getting enough overall calories from plant-foods, you will *not* "come down" with a protein deficiency.

If I were wrong on this, we would not see amazing vegan athletes, running ultra-marathons, and competing at the highest levels, in every major sport on earth. I would not, certainly, at 45, be in the best shape of my life. Plus, it's unlikely we'd have some of the largest, strongest animals on earth – who consume almost *nothing* save raw plant-foods – living such vibrantly-healthy lives as they do. Elephants. Chimpanzees. And so many more. Think of the gorillas, and great apes of the world, who, incidentally, are built nearly identically to you and I. Both internally and in their outer characteristics. What do they eat all day long, for an entire life? Fruits, green leaves, and just a handful of bark, seeds or other denser items. The silverback gorilla is about 30 times stronger than a man. Would he be so on a diet of meats, dairy, and processed foods? Unlikely, I'd say.

Focus your diet on raw plant-foods. Don't accept the animal "food" suppliers' notion that without their products, you'll suffer a shortage of some type. It simply is not true.

Do you feel strong and healthy as a vegan man?

Unquestionably. If you consider the type of workout schedule I maintain, I guarantee you this: there is just no way I could maintain it, or do as well with it as I am, on a diet of animal-based, or processed foods. A typical workout for me is eight to ten miles of running, combined with hundreds of calisthenics; push-ups, squats, crunches, and the like. This type of workout takes more out of you, demands more of you, in my opinion, than any other known to Man.

The results are commensurate, yes. You develop an amazing amount of strength, endurance, and overall core-fitness. You sleep deeply each night. You release natural HGH, the scientifically-proven "fountain of youth" from your pituitary gland. And you develop a "ripped", super-lean, yet strong physique. Yet can you do *any* of it, while consuming animal foods and other toxins? Not in my experience. And, by the same token, when your body is *not* obstructed with all those toxins, you'll find you're stronger, fitter, and healthier from the inside out, than ever before in your life.

For men wanting to optimize their fitness regime, do you have any special tips?

Yes. Callisthenic workouts, done early in the day, are the best way to get fit, fast. If you doubt this, tomorrow morning, wake up and try the following: Rise with the sun. Stretch, then jog in place, briefly, to warm up. Then simply do as many body-weight squats as you can. Keep your back straight. Bend your knees, until your quadriceps, your thigh muscles, are about parallel with the floor. And repeat. After you've done as many squats as possible, with no rest at all, begin with crunches. Do as many as you can. And then, again, with no rest, do as many push-ups as you can. Go until you cannot do another. Then, jump up, and do 15 to 20 jumping jacks, to loosen the muscles. And repeat the cycle again.

If you do this for just 10 or 15 minutes, you'll be a "believer", fast. This type of workout builds super-strength, incredible cardio-fitness, *and* a mental toughness that most will never know. And if you do it, first thing in the morning, you'll have an edge, physically and mentally, that'll put you ahead, in your own, totally unique way, of anyone you meet. Oh yes: the workout burns fat off your body like mad as well.

Is there any special vegan food that you recommend for men who are trying to gain muscle?

No. There are no foods that build muscle. If you're concerned about protein, just know this: the greatest protein requirement of our lives occurs when we are infants. When we are undergoing our greatest spurt in growth. What is a baby's natural food? Mother's milk, which happens to be about six per cent protein. Later in life, our protein demands decrease, even more. Yet still, most fruits and vegetables contain between six to ten per cent of protein. The *exact* amounts needed to maintain all the "raw muscle" you'll ever want. Examples? Cucumbers alone are 11 per cent protein. Tomatoes, 12 per cent. Broccoli, 20 per cent. Asparagus, 27 per cent! Again, if you eat plenty of these foods, and other plant-foods, you'll never have to worry about *any* type of diet deficiency; much less a protein one.

Another thing to note is, many believe, due to the fairly successful propaganda put forth by meat and dairy suppliers, that plant-foods contain incomplete proteins. This is inaccurate. In fact, of the 23 essential amino acids, your body naturally produces fifteen. And the other eight? Kale contains them all. As well as bananas. Okra. Peas. Tomatoes. Nuts. And many more. If you eat like the gorilla, plenty of raw fruits and edible green leaves, spinach and the like, *and* you stay active and exercise diligently, you will *not* "come down" with a deficiency. In anything. In fact, as I've found, you'll likely be fitter, healthier, and stronger, than ever before in your life.

Anything else you would like to add?

Yes. There's no greater gift in the world, than one's own health. Most of us are born in a pristine condition. Then, through a variety of factors, we allow that health, and the vitality that goes with it, to wane. It does *not* have to be that way. I don't care what your age is, even if you feel your best years are behind you. I don't care what your ailments, may be. If you begin doing the right thing, you can improve yourself, *far* faster than most would believe. And most of us, know intuitively, what that "right thing" is. It's to eat the natural fruits of the earth, to sustain yourself. It's to exercise vigorously, each day. It's to treat others, all creatures, as you would be treated.

That's the whole of it. It truly is, that simple. Yet so many have made it – the subject of health and fitness - horribly, unacceptably, complex. I can show you the simple way that has worked for me. You can read my books, watch my videos, which I know - from my own experience, and from that of the thousands I've taught - work, incredibly well, if you follow them with commitment. Yet also, you can begin right now, this instant.

Start, simply by going to your kitchen right now. Once there, throw out everything that is not a healthy, living plant-food. You'll feel a deep sense of clarity and freedom when you do this. When you're done with that task, here's another, if you're interested. Do a 15-minute callisthenic workout, as I described, before. Then go for a run or fast-walk, around the block. This'll get you on the right path, quickly. After that, begin to educate yourself, with either my books, or others' who've succeeded with a vegan diet. You'll learn, and develop, much faster than you might think. Is it worth it, all this? After two decades of doing it, and being in better shape now, at "middle age", than I was in my twenties, *and* after teaching thousands of others to do the same, I can tell you, without question…Yes!

Connect with Jeff:

http://superiorbodyhealth.com
http://thesuperfitvegan.com
http://facebook.com/jeff.sekerak

Meeting A Raw Vegan Powerhouse

Ralf Behn
Germany

Highly energised were the words I used to describe Ralf when I met him several years ago. Actually, highly energised is a huge understatement. Ralf's energy could power a major city! The second thing I noticed was his infectious positive outlook. He's unstoppable! A book about plant-powered men would not be complete without a contribution from the powerhouse that is Mr Ralf Behn. Ralf is a renowned international speaker, health and fitness advisor to youth organisations, corporations and celebrities. He is also a bestselling author, health, lifestyle and success coach, hypnotherapist, fitness and nutrition specialist, athlete and entrepreneur. Early in his life Ralf developed a passion for helping people. He is considered by many to be one of Australia's leading authorities on healthy living, raw foods and disease prevention. He is the founder and CEO of the Australian Institute of Health & Nutrition.

The following is an extract from his book *Unlocking Your Health and Happiness* that he has most graciously allowed me to re-print:

> What most Australians consider to be a healthy diet is more like a bodily train wreck. Clogged arteries go far beyond heart disease, and almost all Australians have the precursors of heart disease distributed throughout their entire body. The seriousness of clogged blood vessels can't be underestimated. More people die from diseases of the blood vessels than from all other causes of death combined. The primary cause of clogged blood vessels is cholesterol, and the only dietary source of cholesterol is animal foods! This is why the switch from a plant-based diet to an animal-based diet has been the biggest health disaster in human history. Many people think, I can eat steak and eggs and cheese and bacon and chocolate cake and ice cream and hamburgers and I'll still be able to be healthy and lose weight.

> You don't have to be a nuclear scientist to figure out that this doesn't sound quite right. It not only doesn't sound right; it doesn't look right from inside your body, and it should come as no big surprise that high fat diets cause a whopping 40% reduction in blood flow to the heart after just one year.

> We think that eating a mainstream, high-fat diet is the natural way to eat. It isn't. Meat is clogging your arteries!

Numerous world-class, super-successful athletes live on a vegetarian or vegan diet, and one of them is Carl Lewis, who reached the top of his career at age 30 on a vegan diet, which he claimed better suits him because he can eat a larger quantity of food without affecting his athleticism. He believes that switching to a vegan diet can lead to improved athletic performance. He's a former American track-and-field athlete who won 10 Olympic medals, nine of them gold, and 10 world-championship medals, of which eight were gold. His career spanned from 1979, when he first achieved world ranking, to 1996, when he last won an Olympic title.

Ralf, what would you say to someone that knew they needed to change to a healthier lifestyle, but was lacking motivation?

It's actually a good question because most people know that there is something seriously wrong with their lifestyle choices – dietary, physically and mentally and such.

Well, we have to start somewhere and a good way of doing it is to take it slow and easy, rather than going crazy on a "ten day detox" challenge, and then back to "normal"! Very few people can switch from super bad to super good over night and stick with it for life. It depends on age and many other factors too, you know, even toxic "friends and family" plays a role.

They have to find a mentor, a trainer, a coach or good friend(s) to make the transition successfully and permanently. Read and attend seminars, talks and watch documentaries until the penny drops. There is a lot of negative and misleading information out there against veganism, that it can shake even the most hardcore vegan every now and then.

That's why I always say leading by example and becoming a leader is the best way to inspire and motivate people and that's what I've done for pretty much all my life, as a raw vegan and even before that in other ways.

Literally every improvement is an improvement – eat less meat, less dairy and exercise a little more.

Connect with Ralf:

www.healthpresenter.com.au
http://www.youtube.com/HealthPresenter
https://www.facebook.com/HealthPresenter

Flying High on a Plant-powered Diet

Roland Lundberg
Sweden

Name: Roland Lundberg
Age: 44
Occupation: pilot
Vegan since: 2001 (vegetarian since 1987)
Best thing about being vegan: it's a complete way of life, encompassing life, love, health and compassion. I have yet to find a negative aspect to it.

What prompted you to make the shift to a vegan diet? How is it going?

I went vegetarian before I went vegan as a reaction to my innate feeling that it was not right eating animals. It was cognitive dissonance at its highest level to pet the dog and eat the cow and eventually I could ignore it no longer. In the wake of my family and friends' concerns for my health, I decided to educate myself with regards to nutrition. Unfortunately, much of the nutritional info at the time was (as is the case today) funded by the food industry and I continued to labor under the misapprehension that dairy was a necessity for good health. Had I, back then, had the wealth of information available on the Internet today, I would have become vegan immediately.

What is your favourite vegan food?

My favourite food has to be the original fast food – fruit! I prefer to eat mostly low fat, raw vegan food.

What are the benefits of being vegan for you?

Immense energy to support my athletic and creative endeavours. I think clearer, I sleep more soundly and I feel happier. It also creates, within, a numinous experience of connectivity with nature.

What advice would you give men who are considering the switch to the vegan lifestyle?

Don't fall for the industry nutritional dogma. In the time of the Internet there is little excuse to be or remain uneducated. Male classical beauty is a lean, muscular body. Look at the physique of an active, vegan male - it is beautiful, lean, strong and agile. A diet high in animal products yields a feminine quality to the male body with higher body fat levels. It also makes your body smell foul. It robs you of vitality. It inhibits high performance (including sexual performance).

Do you feel strong and healthy as a vegan man?

At almost 44 I am stronger and in better shape than I was in my twenties. I run, weight train, do calisthenics and martial arts.

Anything else you would like to add?

Some things in life cannot be understood merely intellectually, they need to be experienced. Veganism is one of these things. Try it and you will feel it, and will know, firsthand, what I am talking about.

Building a Healthier Future

Arthur Pamboukhtchian
Australia/Armenia

Name: Arthur Pamboukhtchian
Age: 54
Occupation: builder
Vegan Since: 2010 (vegetarian since 1992)
Best thing about being vegan: is being in harmony with nature, globally, the universe and with your environment – where you live and who you live around.

Was it hard for you to go vegan?

Yes and no. No because I knew where I was going, yes, because of cultural restrictions, habits, because we live in a society full of resentment, full of resistance and pre-conceived ideas. These things all exist around us. We can't run away, that's why it's difficult. If I lived in a cave it would be easy.

How did you handle the reaction from your family and friends? Were they supportive?

With family and friends I have always had a very mature, respectful relationship. I respect their feelings, decisions and values. In return they respect mine. That doesn't mean they always agree with me.

In the beginning, my mum said I need to have some kind of protein; by that she meant meat. Later on, she changed her mind and she is now vegetarian. My wife and I decided to go vegetarian and later our kids joined us. Now we are all fully vegan.

Is the vegan diet a good diet for a builder and other men doing physical work?

Yes. I would say, definitely yes. When we are having lunch, my co-workers like to eat chicken sandwiches, meat kebabs or fish and chips. After having lunch, my co-workers need about half an hour to recover their energy after having so-called "energy food". After lunch I am ready to go, I don't have any problems after lunch. Even if I just eat one apple and a banana that's all I need to keep going during the day. I don't even need to eat a full lunch.

What do you eat daily?

In the beginning it was difficult in meetings where they serve food as part of the meeting, because they usually serve steak. When I mentioned I was vegan, they didn't know what to do and what to serve me. The answer for them is always to serve meat. I ended up having fried vegetables and herbs. Interestingly enough, the number of vegetarians and vegans has grown within the building industry during the 17 years I have been attending the meetings. When I am asked by my colleagues why I eat vegan food, I tell them it's because it's healthy. One of them told me that they are ready to be vegetarian and that their wife is doing it too. Many members of the builder's association I am a member of have gone vegan lately. Now it doesn't sound as bad as before – either you were seen as crazy or sick before. They didn't consider being vegan a lifestyle choice, they were thinking you were forced to be vegan because of poor health or because of cultural reasons. Now veganism is growing.

On an average day:

Lunch is mainly fruit – apples, bananas, strawberries and whatever is in season.

Dinner can be many different things such as vegetables, pasta, a little bit of fried food, pizza and barbecue nights. It's fun and it's healthy.

Occasionally I have coffee with soy milk in the morning at meetings to be sociable, for politeness sake.

Just listen to your body. We are all different. If you feel you are hungry, eat. You will start feeling which types of vegan food are right for you. You will digest it properly, it will give you energy. You will then know that that is the food for you.

What advice do you have for men who are interested in going vegan?

They have to try. I remember when I was at university, a friend of mine told me he was going to try vegetarian food. I said, "What's that?" He said it's a thing where you don't eat animals. I then went to talk with my dad's friend, a doctor. He said it's rubbish! He said we have to eat meat, we need protein, etc. I went back to my university friend and he said it's fine. He told me that many people are vegetarian, and because athletic men such as Mohammed Ali and Bruce Lee are vegetarian, it will be fine for me.

Best thing to do, I decided, was to give it a try. I decided to try to be vegetarian for 91 days. The first couple of weeks were strange. I understood later that I was going through a cleansing process. After that I felt good, energetic, while doing lots of physical activity. I didn't credit the vegetarian diet for the positive changes. After my vegetarian trial ended, I went back to eating meat. I remember feeling tired within ten minutes of eating a meat-based meal. I thought maybe it was for some other reason. A week later I felt the same, very tired. I felt some muscle pain and the feeling was as though I hadn't slept in a couple of months. After a month of this, I thought to myself honestly, I feel bad because of the meat I'm consuming.

Trying a plant-based diet for one day won't work. I tried it for a good amount of time and saw that it worked. If you only do it for a few days, you are already thinking you will fail. If you really want to give your body a chance, give it some time to see.

If you have any doubt, just try it. Nothing will go wrong.

Anything else you would like to add?

There is a lot of information available through the mass media and in books and DVDs, that is precise and scientifically proven. If anyone wants to try it or doubts the benefits of being vegan, just do your own research; you will discover all kinds of useful information. But the best proof is in observing how your body feels. Based on medical science, our body is designed to eat fruits and vegetables. Being vegan will also bring harmony around you. Your aura will be healthy, you will feel peaceful and your family will be full of positive, healthy energy. On top of that, your environment will be healthy and clean, meaning we will all benefit. We are all winners.

If anyone has a personal question, please feel free to get in contact with me.

Connect with Arthur:

pambs@me.com

"If you wanted to be an evangelist for the 'meat gives strength' cult, and were looking for a 97-pound vegetarian weakling to pick on, you'd probably be better off staying away from Ridgely Abele. He recently won the United States Karate Association World Championship, taking both the Master Division Title for fifth degree black belt, and the overall Grand Championship. Abele, who has won eight national championships, is a complete vegetarian, who eats no meat, eggs, or dairy products."

John Robbins, *Diet For A New America*

2

The Pioneers

PIONEERS. BOLDLY GOING where no one has gone before. They are without a doubt, very special individuals. In this chapter, we have the pleasure of meeting four such trail-blazing innovators who have followed their passion and achieved remarkable success in their chosen fields of endeavour. First up, we hear from author, adventurer and veterinarian Dr Andrew Knight. As a veterinary student, Andrew was responsible for the introduction of "conscientious objection" to harmful animal use in Australian universities as well as helping to establish the first humane veterinary surgical training program. He has gone on to become a world-leading animal ethicist. He also enjoys extreme sports, the subject of his amusing article in this chapter. Next, we have Mesfin Hailemariam, a young man bringing the plant-powered message to his fellow countrymen. As one of the few plant-powered advocates in Ethiopia, Mesfin is truly breaking new ground sharing his passion for all things vegan in Eastern Africa. Successful entrepreneur, Jeremy Johnson, then talks to us about the many benefits of his plant-powered lifestyle. Jeremy founded the first wholesale vegan food business in Australia, supplying retail stores Australia-wide. We end the chapter with another trail-blazing food entrepreneur, Alex Tan the founder of VeganBurg, one of the coolest eateries in Singapore and a leading healthy fast-food burger chain. I'm sure you will feel inspired and motivated by each of these amazing men.

The Hazards of Reasonableness[1]

Dr Andrew Knight
Australia/UK

It all began innocently enough. Some 50 odd vegans from every corner of the globe had arrived to participate in the harmonious exchange of ideas, at the 10th International Vegan Festival, in Denmark in 2006. We'd all been forging international friendships, respecting cultural differences, and exuding sensible reasonableness from every pore, when Stefano from Italy finally cracked.

It was at least 50 feet from the top of the Rabjerg Mile – the world's largest sand dune – to its ever-shifting base. During our day hike we'd learnt interesting facts

---

1   I'm grateful to *Vegan Views* (2010) and *The Vegan* (2013), for permission to re-use excerpts from my previous publications within this article.

about how far this dune had moved since 1960. We'd learnt of its propensity to swallow forests and small villages in its path. We'd even had a botanical lecture about an unusual type of ground shrub growing at its base. We were strung out along the top of the dune, politely admiring the awesome view after an earnest day of learning, when Stefano suddenly threw himself off the edge.

Stephane from France briefly considered his rapidly receding downward trajectory, and followed shortly thereafter. Knowing there was no-one else to represent Australia, my duty seemed unavoidably clear. I closed my eyes and plunged into space. And thus was born the World's first Vegan Dune-Tumbling Championships!

Our repeated descents were duly filmed and studied later that evening on the big screen, by the rest of the festival participants, who then voted on our performances. Prizes ranged from a massage by the lovely lady from Finland – which I secretly hoped to win, to a public duet with our brilliant, internationally famous pianist Linda Gentille – that all were terrified of winning.

After careful study, however, the audience awarded gold to Italy, impressed by Stefano's finely fluttering feet during his descent. The Italians have ever been masters of style, after all. As I watched him being led away for his massage, I reflected that at least I'd not won the duet, which was awarded to France – although Stephane acquitted himself well at the piano, despite his nerves.

Instead I won bronze for Australia, for which I received precisely nothing.

The birth of the Extreme Vegan Sporting Association

At least our efforts had apparently managed to inspire. In the coming days an ever-increasing number of vegans of all shapes and sizes launched themselves from a mountainous dune at a nearby beach. Soon we had women's tumbling, men's doubles, and even formation tumbling. Although Stephane's efforts to generate extra lift with an enormous beach towel ended ignominiously, it was nevertheless from these humble beginnings that the Extreme Vegan Sporting Association (EVSA) was born!

The EVSA was created partly to address the misperception in certain quarters that vegans cannot be fit and strong. Our website showcases outstanding vegan athletes from around the world, including top body builders, martial artists and ultra-endurance athletes. It also provides a summary of the nutritional benefits of the vegan diet, such as higher antioxidant status, which may, for example, speed exercise recovery.

A warped sense of fun

Additionally, we seek to demonstrate that the vegan lifestyle is not some kind of grim and joyless existence, dominated by self-denial. Instead, we seek to demonstrate that being vegan can be fun. A hell of a lot of fun, in fact. Unfortunately, however, this has not been straightforward, because some of us have a rather warped sense of fun.

In 2009 two other vegans and I thought it might be fun to climb the highest mountains in England, Scotland and Wales, in the same day, using only vegan food, boots and equipment. And thus the Vegan 3 Peaks Challenge (www.vegan3peaks.info) was born. Next year, eight of us decided to climb all 15 Welsh summits above 3000 feet, again in a single day. This became the Vegan 15 Peaks Challenge (www.vegan15peaks. info) – notwithstanding that we accidentally climbed one of them twice due to a navigational disagreement. After surviving this, we had little choice but to try to run all 15 summits. Thus was born the Vegan Welsh 3,000s (www.vegan-welsh-3000s.co.uk). To the best of our knowledge, this is the world's first vegan ultra marathon, covering 30 miles (48 km), and 14,921 feet (4000+ m) of ascent. As described in my 2013 article in *The Vegan,*

"Another spasm of shivering penetrated my exhausted haze. My lightweight running jacket had been soaked inside and out within five minutes of the storm's onslaught, one hour ago. Parts of the mountainside, including 150 m of trail just ahead, were now completely underwater, flooding my running shoes with every freezing step. The nearest shelter was several kilometres in an unknown direction, somewhere below these smooth summit ridges. With visibility down to 50 feet through driving rain, I could barely navigate to find our trail. Next to me, Kate grimly hobbled on, supported by Simon. Her old ankle fracture clearly disliked the punishing terrain.

The shivering was becoming uncontrollable, and my movements fast and jerky. I sensed the onset of hypothermia. Another hour of this and I'd be dead, or at least wishing I was. I just had to run to generate some heat. But Kate could no longer run, and neither of them could reliably navigate through the near-featureless murk. How had I gotten into this mess?"

Six weeks prior, a similar group of 12 had first attempted the course. However, Welsh summers are not to be taken lightly, and one of the worst storms to hit the British Isles centred itself 1,000 odd feet above the course. With torrential downpours transforming small streams into impassable torrents, a back injury when someone was blown off their feet by 50 mph winds, and one possible finger fracture, the course was closed early for safety reasons.

To simply begin the course (which started at 04:30 AM) we first had to climb Crib Goch, the most precipitous knife-edged ridge in the whole of the British Isles – in darkness and cloud, which cut our visibility to 30 murky, torch lit feet. If not blown off the edge we would then have to climb Mt Snowdon, Wales' highest summit, rising to 1,085 m. The Welsh summer downpours had rendered the rocks lethally slippery, and my running shoes had no grip.

The toughest race on Earth

However, our trials were as nothing compared to those of certain other vegan athletes. In 2012 British Woman Fiona Oakes completed the world's toughest footrace – the Marathon des Sables. This is a 6 day, 243 km (151 mile) endurance race across the Sahara Desert in Morocco, carrying all of one's food and supplies. Only water is provided – and even that is limited. Fiona endured sand, dust and even hail storms, in temperatures above 50°C by day, with freezing conditions at night.[2]

Fiona also runs the Tower Hills Animal Sanctuary in Essex, looking after around 400 dogs, horses, rabbits, guinea pigs, chinchillas, hamsters and other animals, virtually single-handed, as well as training hard as an elite runner. The week before the race she was helping a collapsed elderly horse to her feet. The horse stepped backwards onto Fiona's foot, breaking two of her toes. Despite this, and a very severe allergic reaction to the metal fibres contained within her high-tech socks, Fiona excelled in a race that broke so many others – virtually all of whom were incredibly fit men.

Not all men have been beaten by women though, (probably because Fiona was not there). One such man was vegan Demetrios (Mitso) Kehayioglou, who ran across the entire Greek mainland, as well as Crete, in 2011, to fundraise for the Aegean Wild Life Hospital, and The Black Fish – an international marine conservation organization. In 29 days he ran an incredible 1,660 km (1030 miles).

---

2   Fiona's race report at www.fionaoakes.com/MdSreport2012. html is about the most inspiring thing this author has ever read.

Extreme vegan cooking and flying bananas

However, the EVSA is not all about hardcore toil. We also aim to showcase how much fun the vegan lifestyle can be – although as stated previously, our warped sense of 'fun' can sometimes be hard to understand. Take British vegan plumber Andrew Taylor, for example. As well as successfully completing the Vegan 3 and 15 Peaks Challenges, in 2009 he jumped out of an aircraft dressed in a banana costume – becoming, to the best of our knowledge, the world's first flying banana.

Similarly, the Vegan Black Metal Chef has brought a completely new dimension to vegan cooking, by combining satanic rituals performed in a dungeon, with wicked-looking knives, vegetables, spices and the occasional axe. Set to heavy metal music, complete with helpful subtitles such as 'aaah aaah aaah aaah aaaaaaaaaahh!' American sound engineer Brian Manowitz's instructional cooking videos became an instant Internet sensation. If you have any doubts that cooking can be a danger sport, the Vegan Black Metal Chef is waiting to annihilate them for you.

A less dangerous past time

Unfortunately however, my own attempts at cooking have proven quite dangerous enough already. I therefore decided it would be wise to try something a little safer. Also theorising that women are more attracted to domesticated men, I decided to give extreme ironing a go.

Combining *"the thrill of a danger sport with the satisfaction of a well-pressed shirt"* the popularity of extreme ironing has risen spectacularly. International championships now exist, with the English recently beating the Australians by having the greatest number of people ironing underwater at the same time, in a flooded quarry. The waters were so freezing they desperately hoped they'd never have to win back the title.

As a native Australian though, I rather hope otherwise. In fact, my secret ambition is that with sufficient training, I might be able to make the Aussie team someday. However Aussies are tough, so I knew this would have to be hard-core.

Accordingly, in late 2011 I carried my mountaineering ironing board (specially chosen for its lightweight mesh construction and streamlined profile) to the summit of Wales' highest mountain, Mt Snowdon (1,085 m). Although almost blown off the summit by 50 mph winds, for a few seconds I was the highest ironer in all of England and Wales.

One year later I've just returned from an ironing trip to the French Alps. I ironed above 3,000 m in temperatures as low as -20°C. A wilderness snowstorm even enabled me to practice survival ironing! My shirts got seriously crisp that day. Unfortunately, however, I'm still awaiting any signs that my girlfriend is impressed.

Seeking warmth and comfort

After spending so much time at altitude, I've promised myself that my next extreme challenge will be warm, comfortable and very well-oxygenated. Shark-diving seems the obvious choice. I'm now seeking an ecologically-friendly shark-diving tour operator, somewhere warm and sunny, because I'd very much like to see these magnificent creatures before they become virtually extinct.

The video of the Flying Banana's maiden flight, along with clips and photos from many other amazing vegan athletes, including the Vegan Black Metal Chef, are all available at www.ExtremeVeganSports.org. I've even included some extreme ironing pics.

Adventurous vegans are similarly welcome to send pictures of their own exploits. All who subscribe to our fun and life-affirming sporting ideals may consider themselves members of the EVSA. All sports are considered, but you've got to be vegan! And remember, momento moro, sic carpe ferrum (remember, you are mortal, and your time is limited. So – seize that iron)! Have fun – and iron hard!

About Dr. Andrew Knight:

Australian-British animal ethicist Dr. Andrew Knight is a ridiculously busy bloke. He is a European Veterinary Specialist in Welfare Science, Ethics and Law; a Fellow of the Oxford Centre for Animal Ethics, which is dedicated to advancing the ethical status of animals through academic research, teaching, and publication; and the Director of Animal Consultants International, which provides multidisciplinary expertise for animal issues. Andrew has over 50 academic publications on animal issues. These include an extensive series examining the contributions to human healthcare of animal experiments, which formed the basis for his 2010 PhD and his 2011 book *The Costs and Benefits of Animal Experiments*. Andrew's other publications have examined the contributions of the livestock sector to climate change, vegetarian companion animal diets, the animal welfare standards of veterinarians, and the latest evidence about animal cognitive and related abilities, and the resultant moral implications.

Connect with Dr Knight:

www.VegePets.info
www.AndrewKnight.info
www.HumaneLearning.info
www.AnimalExperiments.info
www.ExtremeVeganSports.org
www.AnimalConsultants.org

Plant-powered Living, African Style

Mesfin Hailemariam
Ethiopia

Name: Mesfin Hailemariam
Age: 27
Occupation: I work with small businesses (offering

training for mushroom growing) plus I do volunteer work related to vegan/animal rights and environmental activism, especially through YVE Ethiopia. I am planning to develop vegan businesses based on vegan organic agriculture and vegan food processing and restaurants in the future.

Vegan since: 2008

Best thing about being vegan: everything – I mean the fact that I'm living by the values I strongly believe in. Veganism is not just a belief to me but also a moral obligation that brings peace of mind when fulfilled.

What prompted you to make the shift to a vegan diet?

I've been on a roller coaster ride regarding my relationship with animals. From childhood, I loved and respected animals very much. I dreamed of becoming a conservationist but unfortunately joined college to study animal agriculture instead, as there are no institutions in my country offering my dream course. In pursuit of following my dream of studying conservation, biology, zoology or related fields of higher education in a foreign country, I tried to contact animal related organisations like PETA and Supreme Master TV for sponsorship and ended up reading a lot regarding animal rights. After a brief period, I made the decision to use my profession for the cause of animal rights and went vegan in 2008. I give credit to Supreme Master TV for offering me the revelation and continued inspiration regarding how to really love and respect all lives.

What are the benefits of being vegan for you?

The greatest benefit of being vegan for me is the satisfaction of living a wholesome life. Not financially or in any other way but by living in a guilt free and harmonious way. The satisfaction comes from the fact that I'm living in the morally right way as much as possible regardless of any other personal matters. The fact that I'm more or less fulfilling my ambition of not living just for the sake of myself but for conserving all nature in general is the greatest benefit of being vegan for me.

I live in the most sustainable way to conserve the environment, natural resources, water, land and food. It is especially important considering the society I live in, where there is a chronic shortage of food and a great lust for meat and animal products. I am being an example by being a conservationist. I look forward to the future prolific vegan society I envision.

Personal benefits like being able to live cheaply and healthily are those that come as bonuses but are good ones to enjoy nonetheless.

What advice would you give men who are considering the switch to the vegan lifestyle?

I say go for it! Everyone, both men and women, should stand by their moral obligation of living vegan. We're not legally required to live in that way for now, but by thinking deeply and opening ourselves up to the necessary information we'll feel we're obliged to go vegan. Going vegan is not like being pragmatic for an ideology; it's more of a moral obligation. Once this feeling sweeps over you, the worst feeling is being non-vegan. Don't make compromises as it makes you weaker nor concede to the carnist's bluff. I'm here living in one of the most oblivious and indifferent societies in the world regarding veganism and animal rights. I've never tried vegan (mock) meats, vegan fish, vegan eggs or vegan chocolates. I've only tried soy milk and tofu once or twice after going vegan, and have never met more than ten committed vegans in my life, but I am still very much thriving as a vegan.

There are more food choices as a vegan than an omnivore. Even if that was not the case, it is better to resort to consuming whatever vegan options you have, as it is always better than consuming or using part of a murdered body. In my life I've been living according to my values and beliefs. If I was an idealist, I'd be living in a remote jungle area living on my own produce by looking after, not exploiting, nature. I do many things wrong. I've a lot of things in my mind that I want to do that have never been realized. But switching to a vegan life after I learned about it enough was an easy change for me and nothing can switch me back to non-vegan living. Follow vegan examples, keep your vegan friends close, obtain videos and books, and check out vegan websites, etc. Label meat and body parts of animals as carrion and others as body secretions, pus, vomit, etc., because that's what they really are.

Did you encounter any obstacles from family and friends when they found out you were vegan and how did you overcome them?

Yes, in fact always. But I overcome them every time by living up to my moral obligations in a disciplined way, and by proving them wrong every time they question my moves by putting forward the information based on tangible, logical, moral and scientific facts. I always stay informed so I can effectively reply to the frequently arising, usually silly questions and "challenges", by relating veganism to every topic, more preferably, indirectly. Also, I overcome obstacles by being more well advanced in knowledge relating to nutrition, food, sustainable living and environmental protection, resource distribution, ethical living and so on, than the people around me.

I stay knowledgeable and well prepared with answers to vegan frequently asked questions. I am a frequent visitor and follower of websites like Gary Francione's (www.abolitionistapproach.com), Gary Yourofsky's (www.adaptt.org), www.vegansociety.com and Butterflies' blog (thevegantruth.blogspot.com), among others. I am also well equipped with plenty of vegan videos, books, brochures, leaflets and so on that I was provided by my close friends from abroad. I usually use these materials for my advocacy activities and to help people around me who would like to learn more, and I use every opportunity and means to do so.

Family members that had been staunchly opposed to my lifestyle are now gradually changing to more of a plant-based lifestyle because of the stamina and persistence I showed, especially my mother who suffers from diabetes and my father who suffers from chronic arthritis and high blood pressure.

Do you feel strong and healthy as a vegan man?

Absolutely…and more than ever. In fact, I am thinking about involving in body building activities, just to prove the cause we're promoting and to also stay fit and healthy.

Are you involved in any work to promote the vegan lifestyle or advance the cause for animals?

Yes and I am one of the leading few involved in promoting the vegan (abolitionist) lifestyle and to advance the cause for animals in my country.

I have co-founded Vegan Association Ethiopia and am now the founder and director of a small advocacy group called Vegan Ethiopia. I also use Facebook (facebook.com/veganethiopia) with the help of my close Aussie friends Faye Leister and Despina Rosales. My mission is to educate, based on tangible, logical, moral and scientific facts. I'm hoping that as many of the oblivious and usually indifferent Ethiopian and African people as possible adopt the vegan diet, by presenting them with its versatile advantages to all members of the society – human animals and non-human animals.

My ongoing activities are setting up and running a network of Animals' Friends Clubs at elementary schools in the capital Addis Ababa, as well as actively engaging in promoting vegan organic farming methods by offering training to local farmers. I also use many other vegan advocacy methods such as leafleting and video presentations whenever the opportunities arise.

Anything else you would like to add?

I'd like to say that it is my wish to meet many more vegan friends even though I'm trying to "make" more vegans here. I feel inspired and motivated by meeting motivated vegans. And I'd like to one day be given the chance to travel for short experience sharing trips to places where there are more developed vegan communities.

With only a handful of committed vegans in this country, I together with a few of my vegan colleagues are trying as much as possible to spread the word of veganism in Ethiopia. It is of course difficult at this level to work everything out by ourselves. We are very fortunate to have some of our friends from abroad who are supporting us.

Connect with Mesfin:

For those who would like to contact me and maybe help me spread the word:

My personal facebook page:
www.facebook.com/therealmase

My personal twitter page:
https://twitter.com/MEthioVeg
My vegan advocacy facebook page:
www.facebook.com/veganethiopia
My vegan advocacy twitter page:
https://twitter.com/veganethiopia
My future website (under construction):
www.veganethiopia.com
Email: meshagem@gmail.com
Skype: meshagem

The Mighty Health Benefits of Plant Power

Jeremy Johnson
Australia

Name: Jeremy Johnson
Age: 41
Occupation: Managing Director, Vegan Perfection
Vegan since: 2004
Best thing about being vegan: being vegan is the best thing that I have ever done in my life and by far my proudest achievement.

What prompted you to make the shift to a vegan diet? How is it going?

I read a book called *The Pig Who Sang to the Moon* by Jeffrey Masson and realised immediately that I could no longer contribute to the horrific cruelty of factory farming. From there the progression to a cruelty free lifestyle was quick and seemed perfectly logical.

What is your favourite vegan food?

That is a really tough one! If I have to choose just one then I would say Vegusto dairy-free Swiss Cheeses. They are mind blowing.

What are the benefits of being vegan for you?

Everything about a vegan lifestyle is positive and every vegan on the planet makes our world a better place. I never get sick because my diet is good, and I don't contribute to the abuse of animals and humans through the choices I make about what I eat. If everyone was vegan then we would not have world hunger, and global warming and climate change would not be the huge challenges they are today.

What advice would you give men who are considering the switch to the vegan lifestyle?

Embrace it and you will never be sorry about your lifestyle change. There is nothing manly or tough about a meat-based diet. A real man is one that knows his own mind and makes his own decisions, rather than just following convention and doing what everyone else does.

I can do absolutely *everything* as a vegan that I used to do as a non-vegan. In fact, I can do a lot more and I am a far more complete person as a vegan.

Do you feel strong and healthy as a vegan man?

Most definitely! My health improved vastly within weeks of adopting a vegan diet, and has continued at the same high level for many years. I am certain that my health would suffer badly if I returned to an animal-based diet.

I feel very strong physically, and had no issues working 90 hours per week every week for four years when I was setting up and establishing my ethical vegan business. And I feel that I have fantastic mental strength as a result of being vegan – we have incredible resolve and belief in ourselves and our lifestyles.

Anything else you would like to add?

Although it seems like the majority of the world's vegans are women, I believe that men have just as much capacity for compassion and love. All too often, men can tend to ignore or suppress their emotions, and this is not healthy. Once a man gets in touch with his emotions, then qualities like compassion and a sense of justice can surface and these are wonderful traits in any person, male or female.

Connect with Jeremy:

www.veganperfection.com.au

Saving the Planet, One Burger at a Time

Alex Tan
Singapore

Name: Alex Tan
Age: 39

Occupation: Founder and Burger Director, VeganBurg
Vegan since: 2010 (vegetarian since 1997)
Best thing about being vegan: VeganBurg. Need I say more?

What prompted you to make the shift to a vegan diet? How is it working for you?

I went on a plant-based diet in 1997 because of persistent digestive problems, and continued for ethical reasons. But I've always believed it's a personal choice so I don't talk and preach about it. Instead of preaching, which there are a lot of people already doing, I choose to inspire and excite people through VeganBurg. The biggest challenge for me was giving up my favourite comfort food. I used to hate vegetarian food, and would do everything to avoid it. I was a passive vegetarian for more than ten years, until a report on the damage inflicted on the environment by the livestock industry moved me to action.

The health benefits of eliminating animal products are well documented, but the most compelling of all is the environmental impact of a world devoted to massive consumption of animal products. It changed my life in a positive way.

What is your favourite vegan food?

My favourite vegan food is VeganBurg's Smoky BBQ. It's the perfect comfort food as it reminds me of hanging out with my friends and having a helluva good time.

What are the benefits of being vegan for you?

Oh man, there are a lot of benefits. Countless even!
Great energy levels, glowing and youthful skin – I'm
definitely stronger than I've ever been! Going vegan
is the best decision I've ever made! Vegan foods
are excellent for increasing circulation and lowering
cholesterol. It's also great for testosterone production
and eliminating fatigue.

What advice would you give to men who are considering the switch to the vegan lifestyle?

I'm not the type of person to ever preach to people. I
think everyone needs to make their own decisions, but
I just try to be an example more than anything. From
effortless weight loss to clear skin, off-the-chart energy,
and smooth digestion - that's all me on a plant-based
diet!

My advise is to eat simply. Our body is not meant to
be complicated. We have more than enough nutrients
from our basic food intake. Focus on creating a lifestyle
that is meaningful and impactful to the world. There is
so much more to do than just eat and eat. There is so
much more to do than to focus just on diet.

Do you feel strong and healthy as a vegan man?

Going vegan means more endurance, quicker recovery,
less chance of impotency, less chance of heart disease
and cancer. Going meat and dairy-free doesn't mean

suffering deprivation. So yeah, I feel very strong and healthy as a vegan man.

Connect with Alex:

www.veganburg.com
Facebook.com/veganburg
twitter.com/veganburg

"To me the answer is so simple it's criminal and it's just people starting to take responsibility for their health and starting to eat more plant-based foods. It's that simple."

Rip Esselstyn, *Forks Over Knives*

3

The Young Achievers

A STUDY PUBLISHED IN the *British Medical Journal* in 2007[1] found that "Higher scores for IQ in childhood are associated with an increased likelihood of being a vegetarian as an adult". I was reminded of this study when reading the submissions for this chapter from our two young achievers, Luke Duncan and Ryan Mays. They are both intelligent, considered thinkers who make decisions based on their own research and logic and have the character and conviction to follow through on their beliefs. They typify many young people around the world who are no longer content to follow the crowd and are finding their own way to discover the myriad benefits of plant-powered living. Others still are taking the lead from celebrities such as Joaquin Phoenix, world-class athletes such as Brendan Brazier and other high profile vegans. Whichever way they arrive at the plant-powered lifestyle it is clearly a choice that is setting them up for a great start in life.

1   BMJ 2007; 334:245

Discovering Strength and Vitality through the Plant-powered Lifestyle

Luke Duncan
USA

Name: Luke Duncan
Age: 24
Occupation: video producer and health activist
Vegan since: January 2008
Best thing about being vegan: the vegan philosophy compliments my views on the world, and it allows me to present myself genuinely.

What prompted you to make the shift to a vegan diet? How is it working for you?

I adopted vegetarianism in September 2007 after doing some research regarding healthier eating and being exposed to the world of farm animals. I quit eating meat literally overnight, and have never touched it since.

My father purchased some books for me to continue my research, and a few of them talked about veganism. The only dairy I was still consuming of significance was milk, but I slowly became educated about the fact that the dairy industry is just as cruel (if not more so) than the meat industry. I also learned more about plant-based sources of the nutrients found in milk, and my consuming it started to make less and less sense to me as the days passed. My initial thoughts towards veganism was that it was a little too radical for me, but four months after letting go of meat, I let go of dairy entirely as well.

I grew up being out of shape and largely sedentary. My adoption of a vegan lifestyle came as I was learning more and more about how to live a healthy, active existence, and though I can't say how things would've progressed had I not made that decision, it's proven to give me everything I need to build a lean, fit, and strong body.

I know some individuals deal with social discomfort living as a vegan, but I have had a pleasurable experience during my five years. It always peaks people's curiosity when my nutrition habits are brought up. I get a lot of the same questions each time ("Where do you get your protein?" etc.), but most people listen to what I have to say and, if nothing else, leave the conversation with a little more understanding of why we live the way we do and how they relate to the bigger picture.

What is your favourite vegan food?

As far as I'm concerned, nothing beats some good, fresh, ripe fruit. Organic, home-grown watermelon and peaches are some of my delicacies.

What are the benefits of being vegan for you?

The vegan lifestyle has helped me to discover my health and vitality. Along with that, my confidence has grown tremendously and I have a very strong sense of self.

I feel that a proper vegan diet (whole-food, plant-based) allows our bodies to return to a physiological equilibrium that our modern lifestyles offset all too easily. By restoring our health and opening the door for greater physical prowess, we are able to address our emotional, spiritual, and social lives in ways that are beyond the wherewithal of those living the standard-American way of life.

What advice would you give men who are considering the switch to the vegan lifestyle?

Eat sufficient calories. An active, healthy, virile man has a significant energy and nutrient requirement, so getting enough food is a primary concern. Pick your favorite fruits and vegetables (and some additional whole-plant-foods if desired), and eat until you're satiated at each meal.

Calorie restriction applies to diets based on junk food and animal products. Fruits and vegetables have never made anyone fat or contributed to the onset of a disease. Figure out your caloric needs and meet them consistently.

Do you feel strong and healthy as a vegan man?

Absolutely. My bodyweight hovers around 150 pounds (I'm 6 feet 1 inch tall) regardless of how much I eat (so long as they're clean calories). Being a natural lightweight automatically gives you the potential for great endurance, but even so, I'm stronger than most of the men I contact with on a daily basis (regardless of their diet and lifestyle practices).

As a vegan, I have dead lifted double my bodyweight (300 pounds in January 2010) and performed a three-quarter bodyweight overhead press (120 pounds in March 2011).

Anything else you would like to add?

I feel that the choice to adopt veganism has to come from the heart. Though it's easy to argue for the vegan lifestyle on rational grounds, ultimately it's a decision based on how you feel your relationship is to your body, the creatures we share this world with, and the planet itself. The most successful vegans are grounded in their conviction, and we are confident in who we are and what we stand for.

Veganism is often inaccurately associated with weak, frail people (especially among men), and I have made it one of my long-term goals to do everything I can to put that stereotype to rest. Many others are realizing that being vegan doesn't mean those things (or any of the other pre-conceived notions that persist), and it's becoming easier every day to live the vegan lifestyle.

Connect with Luke:

www.laymansstrength.com
www.youtube.com/user/LaymansStrength

The Many Benefits of Plant-powered Living

Ryan Mays
USA

Name: Ryan Mays
Age: 22
Occupation: student
Vegan since: July 10 2011 (vegetarian a year before that)
Best thing about being vegan: being compassionate towards all living creatures, and being free from the constraints of bad health.

What prompted you to make the switch to a plant-based diet?

The initial motivation for my shift to a vegetarian diet was in regards to my personal health; not that I wasn't aware of the concept of "veganism", but I thought that one still needed eggs or dairy products for optimal health, and, like most people, I assumed I could never give up eating those comfort foods that I loved, as well my (flawed) belief that vegans were unnecessarily extreme in their practices.

After almost a year on a vegetarian diet, I was unable to ascertain any tangible benefits to my health; I still felt fatigued on a regular basis, and was still overcome by a litany of common illnesses. In July of 2011, a vegan friend of mine insisted that I watch a documentary entitled *Earthlings*, which detailed the reality of our treatment and use of animals for selfish and inhumane purposes. I'm not given to emotion as a general rule, but as I watched this documentary, I shed tears of remorse and shame, for I was now fully aware of how reprehensible my behavior towards animals had been, with my consumption of them and their subsequent byproducts. In that moment, I knew that, being equipped with this newfound knowledge and education, and being in the grips of my conscience, I had the responsibility and the privilege to make the transition to a vegan lifestyle. I knew that my desire to change would be driven primarily out of concern for the wellbeing of the animals and the environment that we as humans share with them; health benefits were simply a bonus!

Do you have any favourite foods?

My fiancé and I make this delicious dish that I simply call "Jalfrezi", owing its name to the blend of spices that we add to it. It involves brown rice, cardamom, cumin, coriander, and several other seasonings. We add bell peppers, edemamé, black beans, kale, spring mix, or any number of vegetables we have in the fridge! It's incredibly nutritious and extremely filling. We mix all the ingredients in a wok and let everything simmer; to this day, it's one of my favorite meals. Additionally, we love to peruse all sorts of vegan recipe websites for new ideas and we enjoy going to eat at our favorite vegan-friendly delis and Mexican restaurants.

What are the benefits of being vegan?

Being a vegan for me is not simply an extension of who I am as an individual; it's the very essence of who I am as a person. It influences my religious beliefs, my dietary choices, my activism, along with many other facets of who I am. Daily, I'm aware of how my choices are able to impact the world in a myriad of positive ways. Being a vegan means that I have the ability to practice compassion and be cruelty-free, be considerate towards the environment, and possess the opportunity to enhance my overall health and well-being. Participating in a vegan lifestyle has cultivated a sense of kindness and understanding within me, and I believe that it's made me more caring towards both people and animals, along with the beautiful earth that we share.

Do you feel strong and healthy as a vegan man?

In West Tennessee (the region that I currently inhabit), the prevailing mindset is that one needs animal protein and dairy products to be strong, fit and healthy. In particular, many people around me assign gender-roles to certain foods, i.e., "meat is man-food" and "salads are chick-food", and the like. I currently work at a supplement store, and I've had many conversations with my customers who insist that you need meat to be a strong athlete. Subsequently, they're bewildered when I share with them that, in my free time, I run marathons, go to the gym, go rock climbing and hike in the near-by state parks, all on a completely vegan diet! Since I've transitioned to an entirely plant-based diet, I've gained more strength than ever before, and my endurance has likewise greatly increased. I've read the works of Scott Jurek, Rich Roll and Brendan Brazier, along with other vegan athletes, and I've found absolutely no reason why my vegan diet would compromise my athletic performance, through my research and my personal experience.

Are you involved in any work to promote the vegan lifestyle or advance the cause for animals?

At the moment, being a full time college student, who's preparing to attend graduate school, studying has taken up most of my time, and I have been unable to devote much of my time to directly serving my local animal population. That being said, all vegans (including me) should find a way to promote animal welfare at every opportunity.

"Nothing will benefit human health and increase chances for survival of life on Earth as much as the evolution to a vegetarian diet."

Albert Einstein

4

The Scientists and Academics

D R. MICHAEL GREGER is a man who needs little introduction. An authoritative, dynamic and entertaining speaker, Dr. Greger is a respected physician and an heroic advocate for plant-based nutrition. His popular video blogs on NutritionFacts.org are helping a growing multitude by making the latest evidence-based nutritional research freely available and accessible to all. In chapter 4 we'll also hear from the very engaging Dr Jonathan Balcombe, biologist, animal behavioural scientist and best-selling author of *Pleasurable Kingdom*. Dr Balcombe enlightens and delights us with his light-hearted and colourful globe trotting account of his real life journey to veganism. And to round off the chapter we have an interview with young Brazilian PhD student in physics, Henrique Thadeu Baltar de Medeiros Cabral Moraes. Sure to one day join these titans as a leader in his field, Henrique shares some close to home "food production truths" that set him firmly on the path to veganhood. It is indeed a great privilege to have these remarkable plant-powered men as contributors to the book.

Watermelon for Erectile Dysfunction[1]

Michael Greger M.D
USA

A disturbing analysis[2] of mortality and morbidity was recently published in the *Journal of Gerontology*. Americans are living longer but sicker lives. We're now living fewer healthy years. Compared to a decade ago, we live about a year longer, but come down with a serious disease like a stroke, cancer, or diabetes two years earlier. It's like one step forward, two steps back.

The UCLA researchers also tracked one's capacity to function – for example, the ability to walk up ten steps or kneel without using special equipment – and found a similar trend. In just a decade's time, we now live more years with a serious illness and more years disabled, meaning we're living longer in sickness, not in health; a longer lifespan, but shorter health span.

The three leading causes of disability in the United States are arthritis, heart disease, and lower back pain,

---

1   *This article has been re-printed with permission from Dr Michael Greger. The original article can be found at:* http://nutritionfacts.org/2012/05/31/watermelon-for-erectile-dysfunction/

2   http://www.ncbi.nlm.nih.gov/pmc/articles/PMC3001754/pdf/gbq088.pdf

which all may be prevented, treated and in some cases even reversed with a healthy plant-based diet. For arthritis, see my three-minute video "Diet and Rheumatoid Arthritis"[3]; for cardiac disability, "Heart Disease: There Is a Cure"[4]; and for degenerative disc disease, my one-minute video "Cholesterol and Lower Back Pain"[5].

Every part of the body needs sufficient blood to function properly. Cholesterol can clog arteries in our inner and outer organs, causing aneurisms[6], heart attacks, strokes, kidney failure, spinal degeneration and sexual dysfunction. As noted in a recent article[7] in the *Harvard Health Letter*, up to three-quarters of men with cholesterol-narrowed coronary arteries have some degree of erectile dysfunction. There are drugs like Viagra, but they're considered temporary, expensive, stop-gap measures that may have a number of hazardous side-effects and don't get to the root of the problem – the artery clogging atherosclerosis that threatens one's life along with one's love life. Not only may plant-based diets help preserve both, but as I feature in my two-minute video "Watermelon as

---

3   http://nutritionfacts.org/video/diet-rheumatoid-arthritis/

4   http://nutritionfacts.org/2011/10/14/heart-disease-there-is-a-cure/

5   http://nutritionfacts.org/video/cholesterol-and-lower-back-pain/

6   http://nutritionfacts.org/video/how-to-help-prevent-abdominal-aortic-aneurysms/

7   http://www.ncbi.nlm.nih.gov/pubmed/21649979

Treatment for Erectile Dysfunction"[8], one plant in particular may be able to play an interim role.

The way drugs like Viagra work is by inhibiting an enzyme that inactivates something called cGMP, which would otherwise dilates penile blood vessels. Thus, enzyme inhibition means less inactivation, which means more cGMP, which means more blood flow. Another way to boost cGMP levels, though, is by going to the other side of the equation and stimulating the enzyme that makes it, which is a role played by nitric oxide. Nitric oxide is made from arginine, arginine can be produced by citrulline, and so researchers tested men to see what would happen if they ate more citrulline. Their results[9] were published in the journal *Urology*: "Oral Citrulline Supplementation Improves Erection Hardness in Men With Mild Erectile Dysfunction."

The consumption of citrulline allowed for a 68 per cent increase in monthly intercourse frequency. The men were given supplements, but citrulline can be found naturally in watermelon. How much might one have to eat to match the dose they used in the study? Three and a half servings a day, but *yellow* water melon has about four times as much, so just a serving a day – one wedge, one-sixteenth of a modest melon should work just as well.

---

8   http://nutritionfacts.org/video/watermelon-as-treatment-for-erectile-dysfunction/

9   http://www.ncbi.nlm.nih.gov/pubmed/21195829

Although watermelon may indeed help treat the symptoms of pelvic atherosclerosis, it's better to get to the root of the problem and clear out the arterial plaque. Just as Indian gooseberries may help treat diabetes (see Amla Versus Diabetes[10]), it's better to reverse the disease (How To Treat Diabetes[11]). Please see my two-minute video "Our Number One Killer Can Be Stopped"[12] and the ten other videos on reversing chronic disease[13].

About Dr. Michael Greger:

Michael Greger, M.D., is a physician, author, and internationally recognized professional speaker on a number of important public health issues. Dr. Greger has lectured at the Conference on World Affairs, the National Institutes of Health, and the International Bird Flu Summit, among countless other symposia and institutions, testified before Congress, and was invited as an expert witness in defense of Oprah Winfrey at the infamous "meat defamation" trial. Currently Dr. Greger proudly serves as the Director of Public Health and Animal Agriculture at the Humane Society of the United States.

Connect with Dr. Greger:

www.nutritionfacts.org

---

10   http://nutritionfacts.org/video/amla-versus-diabetes/

11   http://nutritionfacts.org/video/how-to-treat-diabetes/

12   http://nutritionfacts.org/video/our-number-one-killer-can-be-stopped/

13   http://nutritionfacts.org/topics/reversing-chronic-disease/

A Biologist's Journey to Vegan[1]

Jonathan Balcombe
UK/Canada

I always considered myself a vegetarian waiting to happen. According to my mother, I was five years old before she started giving me meat. So "born-again vegetarian" might describe the decision I made at age 24 to go "on the carrot," as one of my mentors at the time derisively put it. From my earliest memories I've had a burning curiosity about animals and a deep concern for their welfare. My early career ambitions, aged four, were to become either a postman or a hippopotamus. The inspiration for the latter came from family visits to the London Zoo, where I watched fascinated as the affectionately-named hippo, Nada the Lily, would open her enormous gape to receive a whole fresh cabbage from the keeper. With a series of massive chomps, Nada would reduce the cabbage to mush. Rivulets of cabbage juice streamed through pink channels before sluicing down her throat. Restrictions on feeding the animals were more lax in the early 1960s, and Nada would readily accept various tidbits tossed to her from the public standing overhead. I remember a piece of popcorn, lobbed in by some unusually optimistic bystander, getting hopelessly lost in the complex landscape of Nada's oral cavity. Knowing what I now know of the monotonous, lonely existence of so

---

1   A similar version of this essay appeared in *Waist Away: How to Joyfully Lose Weight and Supercharge Your Life*, by Mary Clifton and Chelsea Clinton, 2012.

many animals confined to zoos, I would have changed my mind about being a hippo. Popcorn was probably one of the brighter spots in Nada's days.

The catalysts for my starting to eat animals and for my stopping again were, in both cases, overseas travel. When I was three, my adventurous parents decided to move half way round the world, from England to New Zealand. With over a dozen sheep for every human, New Zealand at that time ranked first in the world (or last, from the animals' perspective) in per capita meat consumption. So it was perhaps inevitable that my parents – unsteeped in the moral arguments for vegetarianism that have since matured – capitulated to local custom and began to put mutton and lamb on the table. Never a fussy eater, I took to these new tastes with gusto. I still recall as a boy sucking the grease and fat from the "crackling" following a pork roast, and sneaking into the kitchen to find the chewy bacon rinds left over from breakfast.

Twenty years on, when I decided to take a year off university biology studies to save some money and go on an overseas adventure, I was well on the way to going veg. For humanitarian reasons I had shunned veal, and whenever there was a meatless option at my college dorm cafeteria, I took it. Now living in Toronto, Canada, I knew the taste of Big Macs, Whoppers, and Filet-o'-Fish sandwiches, and I ordered half-chicken dinners at Swiss Chalet restaurants. When I discovered cooking at age 22, my favorite dish was spaghetti

Bolognaise with plenty of ground beef fried up with diced onions and green peppers.

I chose India for my destination. My mother's best friend was Indian, and I had acquired a taste for Indian cuisine from visits to their Toronto home, where their live-in cook, brought over from the family's lavish Mumbai home, prepared delectable feasts. Like some half-billion Indian Hindus, the Mehtas are vegetarian. Going to India not only meant I would have a congenial home base in Mumbai (Bombay then), but exploring the country plant-based would be a cinch. By the time I'd purchased the airline tickets for a three-month stay, I'd decided to take the tofu plunge. Looking back, I shake my head that it took me two decades to return to my vegetarian beginnings.

Today, the idea of eating meat is as alien to me as India was when I arrived there in January 1984. It was 5 a.m., and Mumbai's airport was already bustling. As jet-lagged travelers shuffled toward stern-faced immigration officials, a tiny barefooted woman swept the floors with a primitive straw whisk, and a scrawny, pregnant cat foraged in the garbage receptacles. Hours later, as a ragged amputee begged at the window of my taxi, I felt the tightening grip of culture-shock, and longed to catch the next flight home.

After ten days, and feeling somewhat acclimated to urban India's constant assault on the senses, I set off to explore the hinterland. Traveling alone in India was

challenging and never dull. I soon learned to purchase
fruit through the train windows from the inevitable
vendors at each station. I peeled mangoes and guavas
with my penknife, heeding the health advisories
to avoid anything that might have been washed in
Indian water. My travels to nature reserves took me
well off the beaten track. At a rural bus-stop a small
gathering of villagers stared wide-eyed at me as though
I'd just emerged from a flying saucer. But "all-veg"
restaurants were never far away. I soon discovered
the vegetarian thali, a smorgasbord of native dishes
arrayed in shiny metal bowls and served on a large
metal tray accompanied by a generous heap of rice.
Indians traditionally eat with their right hand (the left
is reserved for private hygiene), so these meals usually
arrived without cutlery. My subsequent request usually
yielded a spoon that looked more suitable for feeding
a mouse. But the meals were invariably satisfying,
scrumptious and criminally inexpensive.

My one foray off the carrot was November 1985 when
I traveled with a research team to South Africa for a
month studying bats in Kruger Park. Our encampment
on the Luvuvhu River was staffed by two black servant-
cooks. Our evening meals resembled something from
an Atherosclerotics Anonymous cookbook: a red meat
centerpiece and a large dollop of sudsa – South Africa's
answer to cream-of-wheat – doused in heavy gravy.
Any vegetable that made it onto the plate huddled
nervously at the rim, stared down by a menacing slab of
someone's former shoulder or thigh.

Nature found a creative way to reprimand me for my waywardness. Two weeks into the trip, I became someone else's meal. During a daytime bat-tracking expedition, I noticed that a scattering of insect bites on my chest were becoming itchier. Squinting down for a closer look, I realized that one of the little red welts was moving! Two hours later, with the help of strategically-applied Vaseline, I squeezed four oxygen-starved, rice-grain-sized maggots from my torso. Our South African guide just happened to be an authority on parasitic flies. He informed me that my dinner guests were African skin maggots (*Cordylobia anthropophaga*, translation: eater of men), a species not previously reported this far south. So, an off-the-wagon vegetarian had assisted the range expansion of a fellow meat-eater.

I remember in 1991 having an argument with a fellow biologist on the matter of whether or not human dentition had evolved for meat. I contended that because our teeth are bunodont (a term I had learnt in a mammalogy course and now deployed to try to impress or intimidate my older adversary) and because they also lack the long canines and tearing carnassials (take that!) of meat-eaters, our teeth were meant for eating fruits, nuts and other plant-based foods. Lacking that basic skill of argumentation which says "listen to the other guy," I don't recall his main points. It was a rather pointless exchange, for humans evolved neither as vegetarians nor carnivores. Humans are omnivores. Our teeth and intestines are those of a beast who eats mostly plant-based foods, opportunistically supplemented by the occasional helping of animal tissue. Those textbook renderings of early hominids spearing mammoths and chasing herds over cliffs are biased portrayals. Early humans were gatherer-hunters (or perhaps more accurately: gatherer-scavengers) not the other way round.

If I could talk to that biologist today (sadly, he is now deceased), I would not quibble over teeth and spears. For me, the overarching medical argument for a veg diet is simply that we fare better on it than we do with the inclusion of meat. You could fill a bookshelf with studies demonstrating the benefits of plant-based eating.

In my case, the decision to go vegetarian, and eventually vegan, was never a medical one. I did it for the animals. If there were no other reason than the suffering and untimely death of some 60 billion land animals (and greater numbers of fishes) killed for human consumption each year, I would be as committed as a fastidious bunny-rabbit to shunning meat. On the flip side, the health, environmental and socio-economic benefits of vegetarianism are so compelling that even if meat without suffering was possible, I would remain a dedicated herbivore.

Today, approaching 54, I am as enamored by food (and preparing it) as I ever was. I feel almost as fit and weigh only slightly less than I did as a 22-year-old collegiate swimmer. My main source of exercise is bicycling, which includes two weekly commutes to my office nearby (round-trip 13 miles). I supplement the biking with regular visits to a local disc-golf course, and an occasional run, and I rarely watch soccer highlights on TV without a dumbbell in my hand.

My post as Department Chair for Animal Studies with recently-formed Humane Society University puts me in contact with like-minded folks. I also write books and speak regularly on animal behavior, cognition and emotions. Watching animals is a passion as well as a profession, and the lure of bird-and nature-watching get me into the fresh-air wilds on a regular basis. I don't take my good health for granted. I'm grateful every day I awake for another chapter of the challenges and adventures that make life such a precious gift. I thank Nada for showing me the joys of green foods, and animals everywhere for inspiring me not to eat their bodies.

About Dr. Jonathan Balcombe:

Jonathan Balcombe is the Department Chair for Animal Studies with Humane Society University. He is the author of *Pleasurable Kingdom: Animals* and the *Nature of Feeling Good, Second Nature: The Inner Lives of Animals*, and *The Exultant Ark: A Pictorial Tour of Animal Pleasure*. He has been vegan since 1989.

Connect with Dr. Balcombe:

www.jonathanbalcombe.com

Discovering the Truth Behind Food Production

Henrique Thadeu
Brazil

Name: Henrique Thadeu Baltar de Medeiros Cabral Moraes

Age: 29

Occupation: electronic engineer, PhD student in physics

Vegan since: 2010

Best thing about being vegan: reducing the suffering my existence causes to other sentient beings. In clearer words, the fact that I do not participate in the industry of genocide.

What prompted you to make the shift to a vegan diet? How is it working for you?

We are used to buying meat in a supermarket, where meat is not an animal, but a product which comes from a factory. In 2006, I went to a shop in the countryside, where chickens walked on the other side of the counter. There was a room from where someone went out to get chickens and returned to put them upside down in a machine. In this device, the chickens had their neck cut. My family has a farm of latex. There are chickens at the farm, but they just wander around. I'm used to watching chickens and listening to their noises. On that day, I saw and heard something completely different. The chickens were desperate for their lives. So, I kept thinking: do I really need to cause that suffering? From that day on, every time I ate meat, I imagined that scene.

I did not know any vegetarians, so I started looking for information by myself. I slowly stopped eating animals. Firstly, I stopped eating mammals, then birds, finally fishes and invertebrates. In 2008, I became api-ovo-lacto-vegetarian, and also started looking for the vegan alternatives for products such as toothpaste, soap, shampoo, conditioner, etc. After a while, all the non-alimentary products I was buying were vegan, or at least to the extent of my knowledge. I kept learning about the exploitation of non-human animals, and in 2010 I decided to stop eating eggs, dairy and honey, and finally became a (strict) vegetarian and vegan.

Just explaining a bit of the terminology I use, when I say (strict) vegetarian, I mean a diet without any animal ingredients. When I say vegan, I mean a lifestyle based on avoiding the suffering of animals, humans or not. It is possible for a person to be a (strict) vegetarian, but not a vegan. For example, suppose that a person does not eat any animal ingredients, but buys soap with animal ingredients or soap tested on non-volunteers. This person is a (strict) vegetarian, but not a vegan. Now, getting back to the answer…

I love my food. I don't feel any desire to eat animal ingredients any longer. I do not regret the time I spent looking for information about what may contain animal ingredients, sending e-mails to companies, and looking for vegan shoes, belts and wallets, etc. Many people ask me if I miss a piece of steak. Answer: not even a bit, it makes me feel disgusted. Some people don't believe me. Their problem. They ask me if I find it hard being a vegan. Answer: no, we live in a time in which we have computers, the Internet and smartphones. Information is close at hand. Moreover, never be afraid of being a round peg in a square hole.

What is your favourite vegan food?

I don't really have a favourite food, it depends largely on the moment. Some things I love are lentils, chickpeas, a simple sandwich of peanut butter and jam. I used to miss pizza, until I discovered that it's possible to make (strict) vegetarian pizzas. In reality, it's possible to make practically everything (strict) vegetarian. Of course, I cannot forget to say I love sweets: biscuits, cakes and chocolates.

What are the benefits of being vegan for you?

From an egocentric point of view, the best benefit for me is that I hardly ever get sick. Until I was api-lacto-vegetarian, I used to get common colds quite often. Furthermore, I feel that my digestive system works better.

What advice would you give men who are considering the switch to the vegan lifestyle?

Usually men get afraid of losing muscles and getting weak when switching to a vegetarian diet. The advice is simple: don't be afraid, you won't lose muscles nor get weak. I even heard someone saying "I would become (strict) vegetarian if I didn't have to take protein injections". Protein injections!? Nonsense. A (strict) vegetarian diet provides all the amino acids you need, and you don't have to think about combining food, just eat properly. As far as I know, protein is one of the easiest ingredients to acquire.

If you have doubts about diet, look for vegetarian folks, look for scientific information (Google Scholar is a good starting point), consult a nutritionist specialised in vegetarian diets, and – the most important thing – open your mind to new ideas. "Man's mind, once stretched by a new idea, never regains its original dimensions" (Oliver Wendell Holmes Sr.).

Did you encounter any obstacles with family and friends when they found out you were vegan and how did you overcome them?

When I turned from api-ovo-lacto-vegetarian to (strict) vegetarian, my mother was not happy: "And now, what are you going to eat!?" But after a while, she could see that I was happy with my choice and I could eat practically everything, just without animal ingredients. There are always options, I just had to teach her a bit. I have only visited her once since I became a (strict) vegetarian, and there was plenty of vegetarian food for me, including cake. Besides, I see that vegetarianism is growing nicely in my city.

My real friends always support me, some of them even ask me to take them to a vegetarian restaurant.

I remember one in Brazil who loved to eat vegetarian feijoada. Feijoada is a dish from Portugal and their former colonies made of beans, spices and different types of meat. In that vegetarian restaurant, they replaced the meat with vegetarian sausage and some soy protein. It was great.

"Vegetarian for most of my life, I have never really experienced illness. Now at sixty-eight, several years vegan, I find that I have never been healthier: I weigh less than I did at thirty; I am stronger than I was at forty; I have fewer colds or minor illnesses than at fifty; and in my entire life I have experienced no major illness of any kind. I have never, I am glad to say, been to a hospital except as a visitor."

Jeffrey Moussaieff Masson, *The Face on Your Plate: the Truth About Food*

5

Plant-powered from Birth

THE STRENGTH, ENERGY and health a plant-powered diet can provide is illustrated in this chapter by two exceptional men who have eaten that way from birth. They are both living proof of the numerous benefits that a lifetime of eating a plant-powered diet can bestow. Rajnish Dave grew up as a vegetarian and later transitioned to veganism. Yash Sidhu was raised as vegan and has remained that way his entire life. They are both in excellent shape and will attest to not having experienced any deficiencies or problems with their diet. Their fine examples illustrate that eating plant-powered provides adequate nutrition throughout the lifespan of a human being. Not only are they thriving as individuals but they are also inspiring others to make the transition to plant-powered eating – not least through sharing their cultural traditions and recipes for delicious Indian meals. Be prepared for some mouth-watering reading!

Helping Others Follow a Plant-powered Lifestyle

Rajnish Dave
India/USA

Name: Rajnish Dave
Age: 41
Occupation: HIV/AIDS researcher and LGBT (i.e., lesbian, gay, bisexual, transexual) non-profit work
Vegan Since: birth, 1969
Best thing about being vegan: standing up for animals. In addition, by sharing my knowledge of vegan foods I tell my friends they can make a choice not to put an animal on the dinner table.

I was born in India and raised in a vegan family. The term vegan was not familiar to me until late in my adulthood. Technically, according to the western definitions, my early childhood and my family would be identified as lacto-vegetarians as consumption of cow's milk, yogurt and ghee is part of the Indian culture. Often, in traditional Indian life, when the bride was married her parents would gift her a cow and a bull. These animals were integral to the family and well cared for as important family members. My grand parents had several cows when they were a young couple. After coming to the United States in my late 20s, I became more familiar with the concept of veganism and the cruelty associated with the dairy industry. As a result, I transitioned from lacto-vegetarian to vegan around the year 2000.

One of the greatest gifts my parents ever gave me was never introducing me to animal-based foods in my diet. I have never eaten meat, eggs or fish in my life. I also do not desire vegan foods that look or taste like meat, eggs or fish. From my childhood my parents ingrained in me to be compassionate towards all animals and to practice non-violence and that is my biggest motivator to continue my life as a vegan. Besides my parents, there are several historical figures in Indian history that are great examples of non-violence and practitioners of veganism. Some examples that come to mind include Mahatma Gandhi and King Asoka. Jains as a religious sect have perhaps the most advanced understanding of veganism and I try to put some of their concepts into practice. In contemporary times individuals like Noel Polanco (vegan fitness model), Robert Cheeke and Brendan Brazier are some great individuals I look up to as ambassadors of plant-based nutrition and compassionate living.

I can't imagine a different life for myself and I am proud to be a vegan. For my friends who try to be vegan I love to extend a supporting hand. I always tell them it is very easy to be a vegan. My approach is to share and teach and not to judge or preach. There are certain choices that cannot be tolerated. I most definitely appreciate the work done by PETA and Mercy for Animals, in ways in which they expose cruelty in the dairy and farm industry. We have to be united, take action and stop it. There is no excuse for wearing fur. I will never condone anyone that wears fur. As far as diet is concerned, those changes take time and with patience we can reduce overall consumption of animal based products and thus reduce cruelty in our society.

In a decade I have seen an increased awareness about veganism. Movies like *Forks Over Knives* are game changers. I wonder what the next decade will bring. Yay for veganism!

As a life-long vegetarian and long-time vegan, have you ever experienced any deficiencies due to your diet such as low iron or vitamin B12? If so, was it difficult to fix and what did you do to fix it? Do you take any regular supplements?

I have never experienced any nutrient deficiencies per my doctor who examines me frequently. I have a diverse nutrient-dense diet but do not use supplements.

What do you eat for protein?

Proteins are sourced from soy, beans and lentils, grains and vegetable sources (broccoli, spinach, peas, etc).

How do you feel as a vegan - physically, emotionally and spiritually?

Physically strong, emotionally calm, spiritually balanced.

Is there anything else you would like to add?

It's extremely easy to become a vegetarian or a vegan. It is not an expensive proposition. In fact it is rather cheaper to live on a vegan diet. Much against the popular misconceptions, protein deficiency is not the challenge, nor is alterations in testosterone as a result of soy consumption. I have had my levels measured and I consume a balanced diet.

Connect with Rajnish:

www.facebook.com/vegan0dave

Thriving on a Plant-powered Diet for Life

Yash Sidhu
India

Name: Yash Sidhu
Age: 23
Occupation: airline pilot
Vegan since: birth, 1990
Best thing about being vegan: to know that you are not taking any other living being's life to feed yourself.

What prompted you to make the shift to a vegan diet? How is it working for you?

For me my parents were vegan so I grew up in such an environment. Initially, I followed the diet as my parents did but once I was old enough I realized how glad I was that I was always on the right track, eating clean, eating good and eating as nature intended us to do.

What is your favourite vegan food?

One of my most favorite vegan dishes is a traditional Indian dish – Kidney Bean Curry with rice.

Ingredients

3/4 cup kidney beans
1 1/2 cups rice
1/2 tsp cumin seeds
1 small stick of cinnamon
1/2 cup sliced onions
1 tbsp thinly sliced ginger
1 to 2 sliced green chillies
1/4 tsp turmeric powder
1 tbsp coriander powder
1 tbsp dried mango powder
1/2 tsp black salt
1 tbsp oil
salt to taste

Method

1. Get boiled kidney beans (canned) from your local store or if you want you can boil fresh beans yourself.

2. Heat the oil in a pan. Add the cumin seeds and cinnamon and allow them to crackle.

3. Add the onions and sauté for a few minutes until they are translucent. Add the ginger and green chillies and sauté for a few more minutes.

4. Add the boiled kidney beans, along with two cups of water, turmeric powder, coriander powder and salt.

5. Cook until you get the desired consistency in the curry.

6. Serve hot along with steamed rice.

What are the benefits of being vegan for you?

I feel healthy all the time, I don't have to worry about high cholesterol or any of the sickness derived from raw or unclean meat. I am eating what nature directly offers, the fruits, veggies, lentils and all of them keep me feeling fit and fresh.

I have never suffered from obesity – a problem that half the world's population is going through. Also not something that many people would think of but, being a vegan always keeps my grocery bills in check. Now who wouldn't mind that.

What advice would you give men who are considering the switch to the vegan lifestyle?

Anyone out there who is thinking of switching over to a vegan lifestyle, I would like to tell you that instead of thinking, go for the change. You will feel fitter and healthier not only physically but also spiritually. You will feel lighter than ever and knowing that just by changing your lifestyle you are saving so many lives, I am sure every time you eat a vegan meal you will eat with a smile.

Do you feel strong and healthy as a vegan man?

Heck yeah, it has been working great for me. I am 23 years old, 181 centimetres tall and 80 kilograms, healthy and hearty. I am currently on a strength-training program and with just under three months of training I am already squatting my bodyweight and dead lifting over 100 kilograms and that is without any supplements – eating only lentils, fruits and veggies.

Anything else you would like to add?

I have been a vegan for 23 years. I have never had any vitamin or mineral deficiency or any illness due to my diet. I am fit and getting stronger day by day. Not only that, I feel more peaceful, my mind is always at ease and it's always a good feeling knowing I am eating clean and pure, no blood, no flesh involved.

"If we decrease our practice of exploiting animals for food, we will find our levels of disease, mental illness, conflict, and environmental and social devastation likewise decreasing. Rather than ravaging the earth's body and decimating and incarcerating her creatures, we can join with the earth and be a force for creating beauty and spreading love, compassion, joy, peace, and celebration."

Will Tuttle, *The World Peace Diet*

6

The Teachers

WHETHER TALKING ABOUT veganism in the classroom, engaging in articulate online discussion or simply acting as powerful role models by exuding vibrant good health and wellbeing, the four contributors to this chapter are all fabulous ambassadors for the plant-powered lifestyle. While motivated by different reasons (from environmental activism to beating a family curse of lifestyle illnesses), they would all agree that giving up animal products is one of the best decisions they have ever made. In their professions, they dedicate their time and energy to sharing their specialised fields of knowledge. In life, some have used their passion for teaching to pass on their wealth of experience about the benefits of plant-powered eating. Like many in this noble profession, they are all highly valued and respected members of their communities with an incredible capacity to influence others and shape change and opinion at a grassroots level. Let's hear now from these amazing men.

The Taste Sensations of Plant-powered Food

Keith Allison
USA

Name: Keith Allison
Age: 38
Occupation: elementary school teacher
Vegan since: October 2011 (vegetarian since January 1998)
Best thing about being vegan: for me, the highlights of being a vegan are that every day I feel like I am making a difference in improving this world and I feel more connected to my values and compassion.

What prompted you to make the shift to a vegan diet? How is it going?

I had been vegetarian for 14 years and went around thinking that I had removed the death and cruelty from my food. Then I stumbled across some images of the dairy industry one evening. I realized that I had absolutely no idea what was involved in milk production. I decided that if I was going to support the industry, I needed to learn more about it. I spent the evening researching online. What I discovered was shocking for me. Cruelty and death are not absent but abundant. I went to bed with thoughts of some favorite foods that I would have to give up floating through my head, but woke up knowing that I could never support dairy and eggs again. It took about a week for a few cravings to subside and new cravings to replace them.

People always think it is so hard being a vegan, and it is, but not for the reasons I and so many others thought it would be. Cooking, baking, and finding things to eat aren't hard for me at all. In fact, I enjoy food more now than ever before. What makes being a vegan hard is watching so many others around you continue to contribute to immense cruelty and destruction and finding it so hard to help them care enough to change.

What is your favourite vegan food?

I enjoy making and eating many different kinds of foods. You can't top the smell or the taste of homemade bread baking in the oven. Fresh fruit is so simple but the tastes can be simply amazing when you stop to enjoy fresh peaches, mangoes, kiwis, strawberries, or pineapples. I enjoy creating new varieties of smoothies using whatever I have on hand. Some of my favorite dishes to prepare are General Tso's tofu, Pad Thai, Panang curry, and Straw Hats (recipe below). It is also hard to beat the simplicity and tastiness of a TLT (tempeh – the smoky strips, lettuce, tomato sandwich) with a little vegan mayo.

Recipe for Straw Hats:

Heat the contents of a can of black beans in the oven, without draining the liquid. Add half a packet of taco seasoning. Serve over Fritos (or use tortilla chips) with kale or lettuce, diced tomatoes, onions, salsa, and guacamole.

What are the benefits of being vegan for you?

I have never felt more in tune with my compassion. I have never felt as active in improving the world. I have never enjoyed food and cooking more than I do now. I weigh less than at any point since 1994, when I was halfway through college. I feel healthier and look better than at any point in my adult life.

What advice would you give men who are considering the switch to the vegan lifestyle?

Try it for 30 days. You don't have to feel like this has to be a forever decision. Anyone can stick to it for 30 days. When your time is up, however, I'm guessing that your body won't want you to stop. You will feel a physical difference and you will love that feeling. Your body will talk you into continuing and your compassion will thank you for it.

Do you feel strong and healthy as a vegan man?

I feel healthier than I ever have before and I certainly have not lost any strength.

The Environmental Benefits of a Plant-powered Diet

Scott Garant
Canada

Name: Scott Garant
Age: 44
Occupation: elementary school teacher, American Sign Language and English interpreter, artist
Vegan since: November 2009
Best thing about being vegan: the creativity that is spurred when preparing vegan meals.

What prompted you to make the shift to a vegan diet? How is it working for you?

I am an environmental vegan. Teaching the Ontario science curriculum, which has a strong pro-environment focus, to students in grades seven and eight has me doing a lot of research to make sure I make my lessons current. In doing the research, I became more and more aware of the damage that factory farming is doing to our environment. I initially became vegetarian but as I learned more through my research and become more comfortable with vegan cooking, I became vegan and I have to say, it is working very well for me and, hopefully, my impact on the environment.

What is your favourite vegan food?

Just one? Seitan Marsala at Candle Cafe in New York City is by far the best meal I have ever had and I will definitely be making that one day soon! I honestly do not have one favourite as I am constantly creating new meals with the variety of foods that I now enjoy as a vegan. The cornucopia of flavours, textures, and colours make for a never-ending list of favourites.

What are the benefits of being vegan for you?

By being vegan in all aspects of my life I am positively impacting the environment by reducing my carbon emissions, improving the health of myself and others, as well as reducing the unnecessary impact of the killing and maiming of billions of animals annually. I have more energy, and feel lighter in body and spirit.

What advice would you give men who are considering the switch to the vegan lifestyle?

Go for it and do it now! It is all about educating yourself and dispelling the myths around getting enough nutrition. Get over associating being a man with eating meat (and a lot of the other ludicrous notions of what is "male"). This serves no one including you and mostly it does not serve your health.

Did you encounter any obstacles with family and friends when they found out you were vegan and how did you overcome them?

There are always misconceptions about being vegan. This is no different with family and friends. Mostly family and friends harbour strong misconceptions about nutrition and the incorrect assumption based on years of carnism – the belief that perpetuates the eating of certain animals. With my friends and family members who are receptive, I discuss with them the reasons why I became vegan and why most people become vegan: for health, for the environment and to treat all animals equally – people typically don't think about why they find the flesh of some animals disgusting and the flesh of other animals appetizing, or why they eat any animals at all. It is based on "traditional" beliefs that people believe are the "norm". It is all about education and not in the formal way – education through understanding, compassion, communication and the knowledge that it takes people time to change. Most of us also made that change. I have not been vegan my whole life. I had to change my thoughts and behaviours too and I feel that I am better for it. I have not had to "give up" anything; in fact, it has added more to my life.

Do you feel strong and healthy as a vegan man?

I do!

Are you involved in any work to promote the vegan lifestyle or advance the cause for animals?

I am a member of the Toronto Vegetarian Association and recently ran for their Board of Directors. I include veganism in my lessons, where appropriate, and always leave myself open to talking with others about being vegan. I support local businesses that support veganism as well as causes that do as well. Mostly, I just be the change that I want to see in the world and hope that others take notice.

The Easy and Enjoyable Plant-powered Life

Jeff Melton
USA

Name: Jeff Melton
Age: 51
Occupation: college instructor (psychology)
Vegan since: 1997
Best thing about being vegan: it's cool that I'm not only doing right by animals and the environment, but doing the best thing for my own health and longevity as well. We vegans are having our cake and eating it too!

What prompted you to make the shift to a vegan diet? How is it going?

Initially it was John Robbins' book *Diet For A New America* that prompted the shift. After being vegetarian for a few years and not really knowing anything at all about animal rights, my eyes were opened. I went vegan that very day when I read it. Of course, being vegan is not just a diet; it's a lifestyle, and for most of us it is based on the view that animals are not ours to exploit; they should not be our property, but free and independent beings. Though Robbins' book started the ball rolling, there have been many others who have influenced my views. The movie *Earthlings* and the writings of Gary Francione have been especially influential.

I couldn't be happier with living this way, I feel great and am very healthy, and I love cooking and eating delicious food more than ever. I only wish I had gone vegan a lot sooner!

What is your favourite vegan food?

Tough choice! Pakoras, dosas - really anything Indian, Ethiopian, Thai, etc.

What are the benefits of being vegan for you?

I'm not a junk food vegan, I try to eat very healthy most of the time (okay, so pakoras aren't so healthy, but that's once in a while!), so I don't have to worry much about being overweight or any of the "lifestyle" diseases that even people younger than me eating a standard American diet develop. Also, I don't need Viagra!

What advice would you give men who are considering the switch to the vegan lifestyle?

Educate yourself and find out all the good reasons for being vegan, find some good sources of recipes, learn how to cook well if you don't know already, and recognize that being vegan doesn't involve depriving yourself. For every food you stop eating, you will soon discover ten more delicious things to try that you haven't before! There is an abundance of great vegan food, and it's easy as well to find vegan clothing, products that aren't tested on animals, etc. And being vegan is so much less difficult than many other things people routinely do in their lives, such as raising kids, so don't let anybody tell you it's hard. And even if it were hard, and even if eating a vegan diet was not just as wonderful a culinary adventure as eating any other way, there is nothing more important in my opinion than looking out for the interests of the most vulnerable and exploited sentient beings on the planet, non-human animals.

Do you feel strong and healthy as a vegan man?

Yes, absolutely! I look around me and see so many people my age who are grossly overweight and are already experiencing many health problems that as a vegan I'm pretty unlikely to ever get.

Anything else you would like to add?

Go vegan! It's not hard, and it's the right thing to do, for your health, the planet, and the animals.

Insights from the Middle-East

Talib Ali
USA

Name: Talib Ali
Age: 36
Occupation: ESL instructor
Vegan since: 1998
Best thing about being vegan: the realization that an animal didn't have to die for me to have lunch!

What prompted you to make the shift to a vegan diet?

I was initially concerned with the fact that the men on my mother's side of the family all died of lifestyle-related illnesses. I knew that for me to break this family curse, I had to make a revolutionary change in my eating habits. I excluded all meats from my diet at first. Later I decided to cut out all animal products, believing that that is even more superior to consuming dairy and eggs.

What are the benefits of being vegan for you?

I feel great physically! I feel lighter and am not sluggish after meals. I feel more conscientious knowing that my diet does not contribute to the depletion of natural and sustainable resources. Nor does my diet contribute to the development of a heartless industry whose victims are the voiceless. It seems that my meat-eating friends respect me for my diet. They mention my veganism on the list of my positive qualities!

What advice would you give men who are considering the switch to the vegan lifestyle?

Get informed and do it correctly! Don't assume that eating rice and salad everyday will fulfil your nutritional needs! Include some type of legume or seed in every meal.

Did you encounter any obstacles with family and friends when they found out you were vegan and how did you overcome them?

Fortunately, no. I grew up in the American South, so much of our cuisine emphasizes animal foods. However, my mother was supportive of me and graciously prepared meatless dishes for me. She didn't censure me; rather, she took it as a challenge upon herself to increase her culinary repertoire and prepare some nice dishes!

Do you feel strong and healthy as a vegan man?

Yes! As an avid weight-trainer, protein is a big concern to me. However, I find that I am able to sustain consistent strength gains and lean mass on a vegan diet. All it takes is sufficient planning and hard work.

Are you involved in any work to promote the vegan lifestyle or advance the cause for animals?

Not in an official capacity. However, I do believe that by me providing vegan representation in my family and community, it makes veganism seem a lot more accessible to those who, otherwise, never would have heard of it. I also have a blog (along with my vegan wife and daughter) – raggamuslims.wordpress.com. We use it as a platform to promote veganism. We also write from the perspective of vegan parents, travellers, etc.

Anything else you would like to add?

My family and I currently reside in the Middle East and interesting conversations arise regarding our diet choice. Some of these conversations can be seen at our blog.

Meat plays a central role in the festive occasions of Semitic peoples. So, it could be readily seen as offensive to pass on the lamb chops at a gathering. However, we warn potential hosts ahead of time that we don't eat meat and they usually follow-up by preparing a vegan dish for us. If not, we simply reach for the rice and veggies around the goat shanks taking care as to avoid the meat.

All of that withstanding, the Middle East/ Mediterranean provides some of the best vegan options on the planet: hummus (chickpea spread), baba ghanoush (whipped eggplant dip), falafel (fried chickpea balls), foul moudammas (fava bean stew) and tabouli (parsley salad), just to name a few.

Connect with Talib:

http://raggamuslims.wordpress.com

"A diet consisting of food that has been minimally processed and consists of primary-source nutrition is less demanding on the environment. Primary-source nutrition means eating solely plant-based foods."

Brendan Brazier, *Thrive: the Vegan Nutritional Guide to Optimal Performance in Sports and Life*

7

The Creatives

HISTORY IS FULL of examples of writers, thinkers and artists who have brought brave new ways of thinking to our world often acting as harbingers of positive new trends. In this chapter we meet seven talented men from the creative sphere: a photographer, a chef, an author and filmmaker, a comedian, two musicians and a DVD producer. We uncover more of the remarkable benefits of a cruelty-free lifestyle as these men open their hearts and share their stories. We'll hear of talents flowing in creative new directions, lives taking on an important new sense of purpose and musical careers enhanced with an exciting new edge. There are the spiritual advantages too and the enormous emotional benefits such as "peace of mind", "clearer conscience" and "release from inner turmoil". And let's not forget the food and social aspects: an "exciting new universe" of tastes and flavours and the camaraderie of new friendships formed and networks forged. I think you will be inspired by the lively humour, wise words and helpful advice from these fabulous plant-powered men!

Sharing the Plant-powered Message through Music

IFEEL
Croatia/USA

Name: IFEEL
Age: 39
Occupation: rapper, fitness trainer
Vegan since: April 2012
Best thing about being vegan: I feel great.

What prompted you to make the shift to a vegan diet? How is it working for you?

I love animals. I was vegetarian for about eight years before I decided to go vegan. I believe that animals are not on this planet for us to use. Besides that, we have so many healthy and delicious things to eat nowadays so I really see no reason for me to eat dead animal bodies and their secretions. We can live well without torturing and butchering animals for food. It took me over thirty years to realize that my early eating habits were not *my* eating habits at all. They were the habits of my family and the environment I grew up in. I was actually really pissed when this click happened in my head, but it helped me change and adopt healthy eating habits. I am glad that it happened that way, as it dramatically improved my life.

The vegan diet is working great for me. I'm lovin' it.

What is your favourite vegan food?

I love tempeh with veggies, tempeh with quinoa and... tempeh with almost anything. My downfall is desserts. It's a good thing there are not many vegan dessert shops where I live and both my girlfriend and I don't like making desserts that much. I love my after-workout shake: chocolate soy milk mixed with one ripe banana, a spoonful of chia seeds, a tablespoon of peanuts and one scoop of hemp protein.

What are the benefits of being vegan for you?

1. No animals are abused in my name. # 2. I am healthy, fit and happy.

What advice would you give men who are considering the switch to the vegan lifestyle?

Going vegan is a chance to create the best version of you: healthy, compassionate and fit. Get informed about quality vegan food, though. Don't eat just pasta, rice and vegan pizza. Eat foods that feed and support your body. Be a healthy, strong vegan. Work out. It's much easier to build a healthy, strong body when you eat vegan. Once you feel the benefits of your new, vegan lifestyle, you will never go back to the old you. Type in the search terms "go strong vegan" on google.com.

Do you feel strong and healthy as a vegan man?

Most definitely. In addition to eating compassionately, I eat clean (no junk, no toxins), exercise and take care of my body - in many ways. I appreciate what it does for me. I don't take it for granted. Feeling good in your body is a choice. You earn it, it does not come by itself.

Anything else you would like to add?

If you are vegan, be a cool, smart vegan. Don't get drawn into arguments with people who attack your vegan lifestyle. Shine instead. People will be curious why you're so happy, healthy and strong. After we did the IFEEL VEGAN campaign to promote the compassionate vegan lifestyle at the Veganmania concert I performed at last summer, I got so many questions about how to go vegan – from people who knew me and from total strangers. Practice what you preach and people will notice and maybe even try to go vegan themselves. To all vegans and non-vegans I recommend a great book – *Why we love dogs, eat pigs, and wear cows* by Dr Melanie Joy. The book is powerful.

I have dedicated my music career to shining the light on animals' inner worlds, their emotions and life experiences, focusing on stories of abused animals. As I speak from animals' point of view, I think that the only way I could feel and express their message is from a truly compassionate state – as a vegan. My album *Animal In Me* was unleashed in November 2012. It's free to download on my website.

Connect with IFEEL:

Website: www.MusicIFEEL.com
IFEEL Newsletter: eepurl.com/ig6KA

Twitter: twitter.com/ifeelanimals
Facebook: www.facebook.com/ifeel.sixthsense

Making the Environmental Connections

Nathan Burling
Australia

Name: Nathan Burling
Age: 39
Occupation: teacher, journalist and musician
Vegan since: 1994
Best thing about being vegan: the food, the vegan
community and the health benefits.

What prompted you to make the shift to a vegan diet?

It was a culmination of a few factors. As a teenager I had
never been exposed to the concept of veganism or even
vegetarianism; my parents are the antithesis of vegans.
The Internet was emerging but it was nothing like the
social media world we see today. However, I was exposed
to music and at about 16 I began singing and playing
guitar in an original band (Nabilone) with my friends.
We were heavily influenced by political bands like Rage
Against the Machine, Dead Kennedys and the first vegan
band I came across, Fugazi. Like these bands, we wanted
to write songs that had a message and a meaning.

In my late teens I started studying a Bachelor of Arts
at Wollongong University. I majored in sociology,

philosophy and English studies. Through my studies I began to learn more about the environmental, emancipation and feminist movements. I also studied moral philosophy and remember being asked in a tutorial if I thought animals should have rights. It had never crossed my mind until then.

The more I learnt about these movements and ideas the more I felt that's where my passion lay. I began to write songs about social justice and environmental issues and I became an activist in student politics and joined the Wollongong University Student Representative Council (SRC) as the Environment Officer.

My older brother (Adam) was also involved in activism. He had done some forest campaigning with a few different environment groups. At the time he was living in Byron Bay and was part of the alternative community there. He would often drag me to protests and actions he was running and I started to use my band contacts to put on fundraisers for different environmental issues in my hometown of Wollongong. Adam went on to work as a staffer for Greens leader Senator Bob Brown for many years.

Although I was a passionate defender of the environment I had never put together the link between environmental destruction and my diet until I was dragged, once again by my brother, to a protest against wood chipping of old growth forests. It was held at Parliament House in Canberra.

It was a bitterly cold, rainy and windy weekend. We all camped on Parliament House lawn and very few tents managed to stay up. There were some great speakers there, including Dr Bob Brown and David Bellamy. But it was the other activists who got to me. There was a kitchen tent and you could work for food if you had no cash. I bought myself a bowl of tofu and veggies. I had never had tofu before and I was surprised at how good it was. Over the meal I had let it slip I was not a vegan and even admitted I ate from certain transnational fast food chains. The look on these people's faces! I got bombarded with fact after fact about the evils of meat and I felt ashamed of my ignorance and hypocrisy. By this time my brother was vegetarian. I had not yet made the connection, but I did that day.

I returned home after the protest and felt I could not eat meat anymore. My partner was supportive and we began to exclude meat. I was desperate to get more info and recipes and my brother gave me a copy of John Robbins', *A Diet for a New America*. This book not only convinced me that cutting out meat was necessary as an environmentalist but also as a person of conscience. It also opened my eyes to the dairy industry and I felt I could not continue to eat dairy.

How is it working for you?

Becoming vegan was one of the best decisions I have ever made. It informed my worldview in that I began to question everything I was consuming. From clothes, shoes and even car tires. Yes, some car tires have stearic acid in them from animal products! I have learnt to be a great cook, so much so that my partner and I opened a vegan restaurant in the nineties.

The biggest change was at the beginning because like many young people I ate a lot of take away junk food. Once I went vegan I realised I could no longer eat at these places as most of the rubbish food also had animal products in it. I was forced to prepare my own meals and it was a steep learning curve but it saved me many years of eating unhealthy food.

What is your favourite vegan food?

I love tofu and tempeh and Asian vegetables and chillies, that's why I love this vegan Tom Yum Recipe:

Nathan's Vegan Tom Yum

Ingredients:

good quality rice bran oil or sunflower oil
8 tablespoons of Lamyong Paste (Or similar vegan tom yum paste)
1 block of firm tofu (500g)
I block of tempeh (500g)
1 onion
1 red capsicum
1 zucchini
1 carrot
500g grams okra (sliced and washed, they can be slimy)
1 lemon
1 lime
fresh chillies (to taste)

Ideally, these should be fresh but I usually have to use cans:

1 can of champignons
1 can of corn spears
1 can of water chestnuts
1 can of bamboo shoots

Method:

» Dice tofu and tempeh into small cubes.
» Add 2-3 tablespoons of paste to fry pan.
» Fry tofu and tempeh until golden, add juice of lime/lemon and chillies to taste while frying.
» Put aside.
» In a large saucepan add oil, 2- 4 tablespoons of paste and onion.
» Fry for a couple of minutes, then add all other veggies and fry for 3-4 minutes.
» Add filtered water (3-4 cups – this is best to produce a lot of broth).
» Add more paste to taste as well as lemon, lime and chilli.
» Bring to boil and simmer for 10 minutes.
» Add tofu and tempeh.
» Bring back to boil and let simmer for 5 minutes.
» Serve with fresh chilli!

What are the benefits of being vegan for you?

The health benefits are great along with the diversity of food. I also love meeting other vegans and visiting new vegan businesses. There is such a sense of instant friendship when you meet another vegan; it's a brother and sisterhood.

What advice would you give men who are considering the switch to the vegan lifestyle?

Just do it! It is easier than ever now that there are so many vegan products out there. There are some great vegan cheeses available, also some great vegan "meats" if that is what you are into or need, to make the transition. It's never been easier and with so much evidence coming out now about the health benefits of cutting out animals products, why wouldn't you?

Did you encounter any obstacles with family and friends when they found out you were vegan and how did you overcome them?

Yes, for sure. I lost a lot of friends once I made the change. I was perhaps a little full on at first. Once the bubble breaks and you see the mass slaughter going on it's hard to not want others to wake up. I now realise it is all about timing. I ate meat for almost twenty years and I had met some vegans and just dismissed them. But the time came when I was ready to hear.

In regards to my family, Christmas time was especially problematic. Australian culture is very meat centric and it took a few years for my family to get their heads around it. However, as my brother was also vegan they had little choice. The first few years there were many fights and then to stop the fights we brought our own food along. But after seeing what we made and realising it was pretty easy to make vegan alternatives all of my family members became very good vegan cooks.

Do you feel strong and healthy as a vegan man?

Absolutely! I rarely get sick and if I do I recover fast. I regularly get blood tests and I have never had issues with vitamin B12, iron, calcium or protein. Also, not eating fatty junk food for 20 years tends to make you feel good! Both my young sons are also vegan and they constantly surprise their doctor by their health so much so he now recommends veganism to his patients who are having diet/nutritional issues.

Are you involved in any work to promote the vegan lifestyle or advance the cause for animals?

My current band, Dead Deities, promotes veganism and environmentalism as well as a few other isms! I also use social media to promote animal rights and I get to forest and animal rights protests when I can. I am a supporter of the Huonville Environment Centre as well as the animal liberation movement.

Anything else you would like to add?

I would like to quote Philip Wollen here from his "Animals Should be off the Menu" debate. Do a web search on Philip if you do not know who he is. We have used this as a sample on our album and I think it really encapsulates what vegans are striving for:

"Animal Rights today is now the greatest social justice issue
Since the abolition of slavery
Meat kills animals
Kills us and it's killing our economies
Believe me every morsel of meat we eat
Is slapping the tear-stained face of a starving child
But it is not a rogue state
It's an industry
The good news is we don't have to bomb it
We can just stop buying it"

One day they will be free...

Love to all my vegan brothers and sisters!

Connect with Nathan:

http://deaddeitiesmusic.com

Walking the Path of Integrity

Andrew Einspruch
Australia/USA

Name: Andrew Einspruch
Age: 34 (well, in base 16. It's 52 if you prefer base 10)
Occupation: author, filmmaker, co-founder of A Place of Peace – the Vegan of the Year 2012 winner for Outstanding Animal Rights/Animal Rescue Organisation
Vegan since: 2010 (vegetarian since 1984)

Best thing about being vegan: the best thing about being vegan is eating without the karma of causing suffering.

What prompted you to make the shift to a vegan diet? How is it working for you?

I read somewhere once that there were only two reasons not to be vegan: selfishness or ignorance. That really resonates with me. We either choose to eat animal products for selfish reasons, or we eat them because we don't know any better. The more I learned about how animals were treated in the service of feeding humans, the less I wanted to be part of it.

What is your favourite vegan food?

I am a huge fan of vegan sorbet made with a juicer. Here is how we do it:

Ingredients: frozen fruit in smallish pieces. You can cut up bananas and freeze them, for example, or use summer fruits. Or use a packet of frozen berries.

Equipment: a good juicer that can make sorbet, like a Green Power (which is what we have) or a Champion.

Steps:

1. Set up the juicer for sorbet.

2. Juice the frozen fruit in sorbet mode.

3. Serve.

What are the benefits of being vegan for you?

There's the enormous emotional benefit of knowing that you're decreasing suffering in the world through your choices. And obviously, there are huge health benefits. A plant-based diet is better for longevity and well-being, if done properly. (Yes, you can be a junk food vegan, but you don't want to be.) I walk a spiritual path of non-violence. If you want to live a non-violent life, then eating animal products is simply inconsistent. Veganism is part of walking that path with integrity.

What advice would you give men who are considering the switch to the vegan lifestyle?

Firstly, know that it is easy to do, especially in the age of the Internet. There are tons of resources out there with all kinds of information, recipes and motivators. So you don't have to do it alone, or work it all out yourself. There are so many delicious alternatives to charring a hunk of muscle tissue on a barbie. And if you need something meat-like, there are some very interesting faux meats around. These don't really appeal to me, but they can be a good transition tool.

Second, the whole protein thing has a lot of myth around it. If you eat anything that vaguely resembles a normal, healthy diet, you'll get enough protein. John Robbins, in *Diet for a New America* talks a lot about this. He cites how nutrition researchers studying protein-deficiency have to resort to artifice to create a protein-deficient diet. So yes, you don't get enough protein if you only eat processed junk food, or only cassava root, for example. But it is really very easy to meet one's protein needs.

For some people, it works better to go cold turkey – a "That's it - I'm vegan" approach. For others, a transitional period and adjustment works better. If you still eat meat, start adding one or more meatless days. The Meatless Monday idea is a very powerful concept. If everyone gave up meat one day a week, there would be one-seventh less pain in the world. Once you have proven to yourself you can do it for one day, then you have proven you can do it for more than one day. Drop it gradually so you get used to eating less animal foods, then drop them all together. The same strategy applies for those going from veggo to vegan.

While all of the above is "reasonable" talk, I still think you should "just do it" rather than a gradualist approach. Suffering is suffering, whether it is in humans or animals. Going vegan is a simple adjustment. You don't need to agonise. Just make the choice. The animals of the world will thank you.

Do you feel strong and healthy as a vegan man?

Absolutely. No question. If veganism can work for elite level athletes and body builders, it can work for anyone. I live an active life on a farm of rescued animals. It is long hours with plenty of physical work. My whole family is vegan, and we're doing fine, thank you.

Anything else you would like to add?

The time to change is now. What gives us the right to cause harm and distress to others, and to do it on an industrial scale? Animals are sentient, feeling beings, not fungible commodities. Here at A Place of Peace, we have one of the largest farm animal sanctuaries anywhere. Living with these beautiful cows, sheep, goats and horses who are so intelligent, funny and wise, it makes you wonder how we could ever do them harm.

Like I said before, eating animals is a matter of selfishness or ignorance. Selfishness can be dropped. Ignorance can be cured. Time for everyone to do both.

Connect with Andrew:

Web:
http://www.wildpureheart.com
http://andreweinspruch.com

Twitter:
http://www.twitter/wildpureheart
http://www.twitter.com/einspruch

Facebook:
http://www.facebook.com/wildpureheart
http://www.facebook.com/einspruch

Getting Serious About the Plant-powered Journey

Brenton Edgecombe
Australia

Name: Brenton Edgecombe aka "Vegan Smythe"
Age: 44
Occupation: entertainer and musician
Vegan since: March 2012
Best thing about being vegan: being on a path of action which is in line with my moral beliefs.

What prompted you to make the shift to a vegan diet?

For me it was a very long, gradual shift toward going vegan. In my twenties I was an unfit, slightly overweight, cigarette smoking and nearly alcoholic meat-a-tarian! My first realization of the fact that eating meat equals harming other beings came to me about two and a half years ago when my wife and I went on a ten day meditation retreat which was strictly vegetarian (not vegan!) and the issue was highlighted.

After that I began eating less meat, but I thought that being vegetarian (let alone vegan) would be impossible for me due to my work schedule of continual travel - mainly on cruise ships, which have less vegan options than McDonalds! We became vegetarian for our own meals at home, but were still quite relaxed when we were eating out or even if we had guests.

About a year later a friend gave me a hard-drive full of e-books, one of which was Jonathan Safran Foer's *Eating Animals*. This book was my starting point for much deeper consideration, and was also my introduction to the cruelty of the dairy and egg industries. I was still justifying my non-veganism by way of my traveling lifestyle and a vague fear that becoming vegan would create social awkwardness, but I was getting more and more bugged by it. I watched the inspirational speech given by Lyn White from Animals Australia at Federation Square (Melbourne) and was doing more and more research on all aspects of veganism.

Amid this atmosphere of emotional turmoil and confusion, one day my wife and I sat to meditate and when we got up we looked at each other and, almost simultaneously, said "We have to do it." Go vegan, that is! And that was it, we changed in one moment.

How is it working for you?

I absolutely love vegan food, and I'm amazed by the great variety of foods which are vegan; so many new tastes and ingredients. I sometimes feel I've discovered an exciting new universe! Unfortunately (or maybe fortunately) the switch has made my lifestyle of cruise ship entertainment almost impossible, so I'll be quitting that in a few months once my contracts are fulfilled. In general I've found traveling as a vegan quite challenging and often frustrating, but I think that will change as the demand for vegan options increases.

What is your favourite vegan food?

So many! I've always loved Indian food so I can't go
past a vegan Chana Masala (chickpea curry) or Dahl.
I also love felafels, vegan pizza, green smoothies,
Eggplant Parmigiana, Tofu Scramble, fruit salad, the
odd Bounty Burger - the list is endless! My wife's
always liked the idea of raw foods since reading *Fit For
Life* many years ago, so she's preparing a lot of 'raw'
recipes which are often quite ingenious as well as being
delicious and healthy. The books *Practically Raw* and
Rawesomely Vegan both contain awesome raw creations!
I also love the *30 Minute Vegan* series for all kinds of
quick vegan meals.

What are the benefits of being vegan for you?

For me the main benefit is the release from inner
turmoil. I believe that all people who eat animals
are constantly shielding themselves from the moral
discomfort of doing so and it's quite a strain on the
subconscious. My evidence for this is the rapidness
with which people defend a meat-eating life whenever
they find out I'm vegan: "We've been doing it for
thousands of years", "We've got canine teeth",
"I have to eat meat - I'm Irish" (I'm not joking
someone actually said this to me). People have these
justifications so close to the front of their mind that
they can spout them out quicker than they'd remember
their brother's middle name.

What advice would you give men who are considering the switch to the vegan lifestyle?

Do it. Immediately. Then do a little research on nutrition to make sure you get enough of everything (there's so much great information on the Internet). Let's face it, most of us never did any research on food before we became vegan, and we survived. The only thing you need to concern yourself with is taking vitamin B12 which is not found naturally in any plant foods (except maybe some seaweeds - I think the jury's still out on that).

Do you feel strong and healthy as a vegan man?

I've never been healthier or fitter. At forty-four, I'm in the best shape of my whole life. Physical strength was never a bragging point for me, but I can tell you I'm exactly as strong now as I was before going vegan. I can still lift the same speaker boxes, power amps, mixing desks and electric pianos and it still hurts!

Anything else you would like to add?

Becoming aware of our society's cruel and unacceptable behaviour towards animals has really shaken me up, but the great thing is it's something we can take action on. I believe animal rights is the last social taboo - if you don't believe me, try casually bringing it up in conversation. I believe all vegans who aren't hermits are activists as the mere act of eating a vegan diet is very quickly noticed and can lead to fruitful discussions.

I think one of the greatest reasons why people resist veganism is the fear that it will create discomfort within their social network and some societal complications and inconveniences. This has certainly been true in my case but ultimately I feel stronger and more peaceful. You should be prepared for the consequences of your life change, knowing that your actions are for the long-term benefit of all.

I feel blessed to be able to lend my hard-earned music and entertainment skills to the cause of animal rights and hope my work may help create a better world.

Connect with Brenton:

You can check out my vegan over-friendly songs and comedy on my YouTube channel.

www.youtube.com/vegansmythe
www.vegansmythe.com
www.facebook.com/vegansmythe

Chef Shane Discusses the Importance of Waste Reduction

Shane Jordan
UK

Name: Shane Jordan
Age: 27
Occupation: chef and food education practitioner

Vegan since: 2006
Best thing about being vegan: the best thing
about being a vegan is the knowledge you gain from
knowing what is actually in your food.

What prompted you to make the shift to a vegan diet? How is it working for you?

It was not a conscious choice. I became a vegetarian
for health reasons. I felt that meat (red meat and pork
in particular) was weighing me down and reducing
my mobility. I was playing a lot of sport at the time,
so I wanted to feel lighter on my feet and more agile.
When I slowly began to substitute meat for other
protein rich products, I felt lighter and more informed
about what I was eating. As for veganism, I stumbled
across it by accident. I started to stray away from
dairy products because I used to always work with
cheese. I worked in a pizza place and became sick of
seeing the sight of cheese. I stopped eating cheese
gradually and changed from whole milk and semi-
skimmed milk to soya and other milk alternatives. I
never had any idea there were different types of milk,
so this was very educational for me. As for cheese, I
just stopped eating dairy cheese and discovered vegan
cheese instead. I was technically a vegan, but because
I wasn't aware of the word vegan, I just thought I was
a vegetarian who didn't eat dairy products. I happen
to watch a cooking programme that spoke about
"vegans" and I soon discovered I was one.

What is your favourite vegan food?

I try to stay away from labelling the food "vegan" so I just call it good food that happens to be vegan. I love pasta, pizza, curried pancakes (a recipe of mine) and Jamaican patties.

What are the benefits of being vegan for you?

The key thing for me is my health. When I switched to a dairy substitute I felt better internally. My skin felt better, I had more energy and I felt lighter. Of course, you can gain weight eating any type of diet, but the key thing is eating as healthy as you can.

What advice would you give men who are considering the switch to the vegan lifestyle?

I would say take your time and research things before you buy anything. Being a "vegan" can be daunting without the correct information. Do your best to avoid animal products, and know this is not a contract you have to abide by. Take things at your own pace and don't be forced by anyone. The lifestyle is simply about making consciously informed decisions about food, clothes or other accessories.

Do you feel strong and healthy as a vegan man?

I feel fine. Remember, like any diet you can eat a so-called "junk food" way or a "healthy" way. If you eat chips and vegan chocolate everyday then "technically" you are eating vegan, but not that healthy. If you're eating a balanced diet then you will feel better and stronger.

Anything else you would like to add?

Veganism is such a big word, and there are many different reasons why people become one. For me, I call myself a vegetarian because vegetarianism is an umbrella term for different diets – that diet being a lacto-ovo vegetarian, raw food vegan etc. I am a vegetarian, but my diet is vegan because of my philosophy. I want to eat without using animals. I like the fact that we can eat so many different meals from vegetables and not have to eat an animal or her milk. Everyone has their own reasons why they make the move from a lacto-ovo vegetarian to a vegan. Just know your reason and slowly make alterations in your life. The biggest thing about being a vegan is not what food you can eat, but being around friends, family and other people at work who may feel differently. The word has such a negative stigma attached to it. When people hear it they picture extremism and anarchy based on it being linked with animal rights. That can be a shock, and explaining yourself can be difficult too. I have had to explain to too many people why I am vegan, that's why I say vegetarian because at times it can be boring to explain it over again and over again.

As a chef, I specialise in cooking waste reducing recipes using vegetable and fruit skins to make unique meals. My "food wasted" philosophy is based on not wasting food. It shocks me to see how many people throw away perfectly good food. Food waste is becoming an epidemic, and people can do their part to reduce it. I feel people should be more conscious of what they throw away, just as they are with what they eat. If you have leftover food then you should consider doing two things: make a meal from it, or put it in your compost bin and recycle your food. This way your food is being used in the right way, instead of creating problems by combining your food waste with your general waste in one bin.

Connect with Shane:

http://england.lovefoodhatewaste.com

The Benefits of Plant-powered Food for Everyone

Phivo Christodoulou
Cyprus/Australia

Name: Phivo Christodoulou
Age: 31
Occupation: video producer and owner of Augustine Approved
Vegan since: 2012
Best thing about being vegan: I can now enjoy life without negatively affecting the lives of others.

What prompted you to make the shift to a vegan diet? How is it working for you?

There were a number of contributing factors that prompted me to make the shift to a vegan diet. In

August 2011 I was encouraged by a friend to go vegetarian while training for an upcoming martial arts bout. Although I occasionally had seafood during that time, I was blown away at the increase in energy levels and recovery. Sure I would get tired during intense exercise but it wasn't the same kind of tired – I no longer hit a wall like I had for years and I could keep going. Simultaneously I was developing human grade organic food for dogs and I was astounded at the difference vegan ingredients were making to canines.

The deeper I delved and the more time I spent in the company of new friends that happened to be vegan, the more I learned about myself and I felt the urge to practise the love for animals that I preach.

What is your favourite vegan food?

My favourite vegan food would have to be the Vegie Head tacos and Mexi-rice and bean burritos with spicy sweet potatoes from www.vegiehead.com. I am a big Vegie Head fan and I don't think I could have gone vegan without the help of Adele's recipes – I practically live off her recipes.

What are the benefits of being vegan for you?

To me the benefits of being vegan include a clearer conscience and improved health and fitness. I love that when somebody turns vegan they start being part of the solution rather than being part of the problem.

What advice would you give men who are considering the switch to the vegan lifestyle?

What advice would I give to men considering the switch to a vegan lifestyle? Hmm… Do your homework and know how to eat right. It may be tough for the first couple of months as your body may initially dislike the change but push through it – it gets so much better! You may relapse and eat meat on the odd occasion out of desperation due to lack of options but eventually something will click over in your mind and you won't be able to go there again. Whether it is for the love of animals or for the love of your own health – there is a different reason for everyone that motivates them to go vegan.

Do you feel strong and healthy as a vegan man?

Without a doubt I now feel stronger and healthier than ever before. At thirty-one, I can push my body to places that I could never have come close to in my early twenties.

Anything else you would like to add?

We live in a society where many people have an "all-or-nothing" mentality. My goal is to encourage others to reduce the consumption of meat for themselves and their companion animals. Even if you reduce the amount of times per week that you eat meat and dairy – that is something positive. Any change is better than no change and remember that no disease or illness was ever cured with a steak.

Connect with Phivo:

Website: www.augustineapproved.com
Facebook (personal): www.facebook.com/
augustinetheboxer
Facebook: www.facebook.com/augustineapproved

My Compassionate Plant-powered Journey

Simon Watts
Australia

Name: Simon Watts
Age: 34
Occupation: photographer
Vegan since: 2010
Best thing about being vegan: living true to my
values of kindness and compassion for all beings.

What prompted you to make the shift to a vegan diet? How is it working for you?

The HBO documentary *Death on a Factory Farm* ignited
my awareness of animal exploitation and I have been
vegan since watching it. Going vegan is the best
decision I've ever made.

What is your favourite vegan food?

Fresh, organic raw fruits and veggies.

What are the benefits of being vegan for you?

Being a wholefood-eating vegan is better for my health, the environment and most importantly the animals.

What advice would you give men who are considering the switch to the vegan lifestyle?

Engage your empathy. Educate yourself about animal rights and open your mind to change. Have the courage and conviction to go vegan and stand up for what you believe in. Be a protector of the vulnerable. Be the kind and compassionate change you want to see in the world.

Do you feel strong and healthy as a vegan man?

I'm the strongest and healthiest I've ever been and loving it!

"The beef industry has contributed to more American deaths than all the wars of this century, all natural disasters, and all automobile accidents combined. If beef is your idea of 'real food for real people,' you'd better live real close to a real good hospital."

Neal D. Barnard, MD, *President, Physicians Committee for Responsible Medicine*

8

Plant-powered for the Animals

IN THIS FINAL chapter we'll hear from six very special men who talk about how their love for animals has driven their decision to live a plant-powered lifestyle. For these men the primary motivation is compassion and ethics. Not afraid to show they care, these plant-powered champions take every opportunity to be the voice for animals in need. In the process, they gain the admiration of women, the respect of like-minded men and the eternal gratitude of the voiceless beings whose lives and rights they valiantly defend. Our world is certainly a kinder place thanks to the efforts of these heroes in stirring our compassion and awakening us to higher values and a more enlightened understanding of our relationship with animals.

Inspiring Leadership Helps Others Join the Plant-powered Lifestyle

Ronny Prasad
Australia

Name: Ronny Prasad
Age: 34
Occupation: author and speaker
Vegan since: 2009
Best thing about being vegan: my favourite part about being a vegan is knowing that I have the awareness to choose a diet and lifestyle which is beneficial to the animals, to the planet, and to my health!

What prompted you to make the shift to a vegan diet? How is it working for you?

I turned vegetarian when I was 17 years of age. I was walking in Melbourne City and I witnessed a PETA demonstration where they had placed dead battery farmed chickens at the door of a KFC store. After 14 years of being a vegetarian, I decided to get actively involved in animal rights. Although I consumed minimum dairy products and no eggs at the time, I thought that a lacto-vegetarian diet was the way to go! I started volunteering for Vegetarian Victoria (a not-for-profit organisation that promotes veganism as a healthy and compassionate lifestyle). Through Vegetarian Victoria, I was able to clearly see the cruelty to animals aspect in the dairy industry. That was the tipping point for me, and I became a proud vegan! Having been a vegan for three years, I have zero intention of going back to consuming animal products. My vegan diet is working wonders for me because I focus on eating healthy vegan foods!

What is your favourite vegan food?

I wish that I had a plain and simple answer to this question. There are many vegan dishes that I enjoy. I do love my salads, and I also love my carbohydrate rich foods. So, I will have to go for a rice salad, with lots of green leafy vegetables. I also eat fruits all day long. My favourite fruit is the humble banana!

What advice would you give men who are considering the switch to the vegan lifestyle?

Becoming a vegan is more psychological than it is anything else (in my opinion). Working in the field of human behaviour, I have found that we make things as hard as we want, or we make things as easy as we want. If you are considering becoming a vegan, and you think that it will be very hard, guess what? You will be right! If you think that it will be a smooth transition, then you will make it a smooth transition. Have a support network around you, and use existing vegans as a resource. I have mentored 12 (as at October, 2012) new vegans through Animal Liberation Victoria's initiative, The Vegan Easy Challenge, and my message to all my mentees has been the same – with the right support network and resources, your transition to veganism will be smooth and enjoyable. If you think that your diet will be "missing" certain foods that vegans do not eat, all you have to do is replace it with something healthy and delicious. Vegan food is to be enjoyed!

Did you encounter any obstacles with family and friends when they found out you were vegan and how did you overcome them?

When I became vegetarian at age 17, my parents were very supportive. My dad had been a vegetarian (lacto) for five years at the time and my mum is a third generation vegetarian (lacto). So, the support that I received from my parents made my transition to vegetarianism easier. Then, I became vegan, and some of my family and friends were concerned about my health (with love of course). My goal was to become a role model by proving to people around me that I can be fit and healthy on a vegan diet! Three years on, I have done just that. I do intense aerobic and anaerobic exercise seven times a week, and feel vibrant, energetic, and healthy! The biggest myth that I have heard is that we "need" to eat meat! My response to that claim is that if meat was a necessity, all the vegans in the world would be dead right now!

You are an active animal activist in Melbourne, Australia. Can you please tell us a bit about your work?

Yes, I am very heavily involved with the animal rights movement in Australia. I just returned from Sydney, where I was a speaker at the Australian Animal Activist

Forum (October 2012). My passion for animal rights stems from my childhood. I have always had empathy for the animals. When I was at university, I sponsored two bears in Asia (through WSPA). That was my very first step in animal activism.

Once I became vegan, I decided to be on the front line of animal activism, and I started volunteering for Edgar's Mission Animal Sanctuary, Animals Australia, Animal Liberation Victoria, and the Lost Dogs' Home. Being a professional speaker, I figured that I could use my speaking skills to be the voice for the animals. Hence, you will find me as a speaker or MC for various animal rights or vegan events in Melbourne.

In addition to the organisations mentioned above, I also support Soi Dog Foundation, The Coalition For The Protection Of Race Horses, Coalition Against Duck Shooting and Melbourne Pig Save Campaign. It is my passion to be involved with animal rights organisations and animal rights events. I thoroughly enjoy it, and I have met so many empowering and enlightening people through the animals rights and vegan community.

What is your vision for the future in regards to the vegan movement?

My vision and mission is to do more activism work for the animals in the future. The power of social media these days is a very potent tool in spreading the message about animal rights. If we can make one person aware, and that person shares their awareness with another person, the ripple effect would be very productive for the animals. Veganism (in my opinion) is here to stay. We keep hearing and reading about the increase in health problems that are directly linked to animal products. Sustainability of the environment is another cause that will help propel veganism forward.

Is there anything else you would like to add?

Veganism is not just a diet or a lifestyle, it is a mindset. A mindset which dictates your choices on a daily basis. Choices which stem from compassion, empathy, and awareness.

If your vision is to see a fulfilling future for the generations to come, then please do consider the choices that you make on a daily basis, and what impact these choices are having on your health and on the planet!

Thank you.

Connect with Ronny:

Ronny's book *Welcome To Your Life* supports the animal charity, Edgar's Mission.
Find out more about Ronny and his book at: www.b1g1.com/buy1give1/book-that-gives
Email Ronny at ron@impetussuccess.com.au

Aligning Values with Actions

Gary Smith
USA

Name: Gary Smith
Age: 45
Occupation: co-founder of Evolotus PR
Vegan since: March 3 2007
Best thing about being vegan: the best thing about being vegan is knowing that my values of justice, fairness and equality are in alignment with my actions. It is empowering to live up to one's values.

What prompted you to make the shift to a vegan diet? How is it working for you?

The first time I went vegan was in college at the age of 23. I had started working out pretty seriously with a friend who had given up red meat to look more cut and defined. I eventually stopped eating red meat as well and became interested in diets and weightlifting.

Late one night on the radio, I heard about a book that sounded interesting. The next day, I went out and bought the book. The book was *Diet For a New America* by John Robbins. I remember turning the first few pages and seeing the photographs of animals in cages, in factory farms. In that moment, I went vegan. I had no idea what I was going to eat, but knew that I could not support the brutality and violence that I had awoken to. Mind you that this was before the Internet, so I had no idea what I was doing. Luckily, there was a health food store and I was able to find food to eat, not to mention living off of bean burritos at Taco Bell and Del Taco. I ate a vegan diet for three and a half years before sadly going back to eating fish, dairy and eggs. Though I went vegan for animals, I didn't fully understand the larger philosophy of veganism, which includes clothing, entertainment and animal testing.

I probably continued eating fish, dairy and eggs for about ten years. There was always this voice in the back of my head telling me that what I was doing was wrong. The voice grew louder and about seven years ago I gave up fish, a few months later dairy and eggs. I think I told myself at the time that I wanted to see what it would be like to eat a vegan diet again, not fully committing to it. After a day or two, I had this peaceful feeling come over me. I knew that I would never consume animal products again. That was six years ago.

What was different this time is that I jumped into veganism with full force. I pored over books, websites, etc., wanting to fully understand veganism. I also became extremely outspoken and have dedicated not only my life to activism, but also co-founded a public relations agency with my wife, Evolotus PR, where the majority of our work is for animal rights/ protection non-profits, campaigns, and vegan-themed documentary films and books.

What is your favourite vegan food?

That's really hard to say. I really love food and the array of dishes, vegetables, soy and gluten meats, are quite amazing. Among the veggie meats, I am a huge fan of the Match Meat products. My wife and I love to use their soy crab and make crab cakes. I love Field Roast sausages as well as their deli slices. I'm also a fan of tempeh, seitan and tofu. We also enjoy making plant-based artisan cheeses.

What are the benefits of being vegan for you?

The single greatest benefit for me is to feel like I have found meaning in my life. I feel like I awoke from a life where I was powerless and without any real direction toward making the world a more just place. Fighting for the rights of animals to be considered moral entities, fighting to end the violence and injustice they experience, doing meaningful work with our business to expose and educate the media and the greater public about these issues brings me deep satisfaction.

What advice would you give men who are considering the switch to the vegan lifestyle?

Do it and do it now. Making the choice to be vegan is the single most empowering decision you can make. No other decision has such far-reaching consequences in the world. Not only are you removing yourself from systems of exploitation towards animals, but you are also removing yourself from systems that exploit other humans and the environment. The amount of soy, wheat and corn being fed to fatten up animals for meat, dairy and eggs is obscene when close to one billion people are starving to death. The single most exploitive industries in the West are in factory farms and slaughterhouses. Not only are these the most dangerous jobs, but they are also exploitive of the poor and undocumented workers. Animal agriculture is also the largest polluter of the air, water and land and the number one emitter of greenhouse gases.

Removing yourself from animal exploitation means you remove yourself from all of the above.

Do you feel strong and healthy as a vegan man?

I'm 45 years old and still lift weights, take my dogs for walks for a total of 40 minutes a day, while being born with cerebral palsy, a neurological disease that causes me to walk with an extreme limp. My cholesterol, blood pressure and other markers are fantastic, especially when most of my non-vegan friends are on cholesterol-lowering drugs.

Anything else you would like to add?

Veganism is the most selfless choice you can make. Like all selfless acts, there are immeasurable benefits that come from giving. By removing oneself from systems of exploitation and oppression, you gain a sense of peace, a deep connection to animals and the ability to live in alignment with your values.

Connect with Gary:

Evolotus PR: http://www.evolotuspr.com
Evolotus PR FB page: https://www.facebook.com/
Evolotus
Evolotus PR Twitter: https://twitter.com/Evolotus
The Thinking Vegan: http://thethinkingvegan.com
The Thinking Vegan FB page: https://www.facebook.
com/TheThinkingVegan
The Thinking Vegan Twitter: https://twitter.com/
ThinkingVegan

The True Meaning of Masculinity

Leslie Jon Heldzingen
Australia

Name: Leslie Jon Heldzingen
Age: 40
Occupation: after sales inventory administrator
Vegan since: 1995
Best thing about being vegan: not exploiting
animals with my stomach.

What prompted you to make the shift to a vegan diet? How is it working for you?

Other than the many, many obvious reasons, one being forced to visit a shop when I was young that had dead animal carcasses lying about. This is an establishment commonly known as a butcher shop. From finding it cruel then to stopping fellow kids in the playground torturing some poor animal, all this cruelty accumulated to the big turning point in 1991 when I was eating a frozen ham and cheese pizza. Just seeing those diced meat chunks hanging off my plate and knowing they were from some poor dead pig finally compelled me to go "vego" in 1991 until transitioning to the vegan lifestyle in 1995.

What is your favourite vegan food?

Apples. No, really. Apples, I really love apples!

What are the benefits of being vegan for you?

Socialising with others of my kind. There's nothing greater than meeting people who condone and practice veganism. Great people too.

What advice would you give men who are considering the switch to the vegan lifestyle?

"What is it to be a man?" is the imperative question that must be asked of yourself no matter how strange it may sound. "To be a man is to be one with the universe". Culturally and for reasons of survival I understand why animals were used in the past when food in the winter months would become scarce, it was either eat meat or starve to death in some cases. So I can understand on survival grounds but when now in this day and age I ask an omnivore friend to come to a vegan restaurant with me sometimes mysteriously their voice will lower an octave and say, "I gotta have meat in my stomach". Men must prove themselves, to prove their masculinity, not by eating meat, not by drinking beer, not by scratching themselves in inappropriate places in public (guilty of the last two), but by respecting all life and understanding that a vegan diet brings us closer to the oneness.

Do you feel strong and healthy as a vegan man?

Yes. I recommend green smoothies every morning (don't forget to rotate your greens), they give me a better burn at the gym (overlook the irony of it). Leafy greens, fruits, nuts, legumes and grains have proteins, phytochemicals, vitamins and minerals that have a direct relationship with our bodies for all-round nutrition and health. You will then understand that a healthy vegan diet is the ultimate human diet.

As Hippocrates said "Let food be thy medicine and medicine be thy food".

Anything else you would like to add?

No...well, maybe, yes...be against the initiation of violence, respect all life and be at "one with the universe"...unless you're eating meat, then we might have to have a talk.

Connect with Leslie:

leslie@heldzingen.com
www.facebook.com/leslie.heldzingen

Making the Compassionate Choice for Animals

Josh Neimark
USA

Name: Josh Neimark
Age: 39
Occupation: website designer and developer, interactive marketing consultant
Vegan since: March 5 2010 (will never...ever... ever...go back)
Best thing about being vegan: my practice of veganism allows my existence to be far more palatable.

What is your favourite vegan food?

Although my favorites vary, in part based upon time of year and local produce available, I am always craving my homemade soft serve ice cream. I call this one my "breakfast sundae", although I typically crave this treat in the evening. Frozen banana, raw cacao or carob powder and non-GMO almond milk. Blend ingredients until smooth. I top mine with a variety of items dependent upon my mood, but it often includes: raisins, raw cacao nibs, organic unsweetened banana chips, fresh berries and some raw almonds or cashews. This is a healthful, no sugar added extravagance, which you never have to feel guilty about eating.

What are the benefits of being vegan for you?

Most people assume the benefits of my veganism are health related. Although that is part of what drives my commitment to this lifestyle, after the first year of being vegan, I found that my interests were aligned primarily with regards to animal cruelty and the environment. The health benefits are a bonus. However, on that front, and after years of training in a variety of disciplines, my strength, stamina and balance have never been better.

What advice would you give men who are considering the switch to the vegan lifestyle?

We created the tagline for our organization – Human by Chance…Vegan by Choice. That pretty much encapsulates my feelings on approaching a vegan lifestyle. My advice is put aside all the preconceptions, look for the logic and "feel" the difference – both physically and emotionally. The time to debate the long-standing arguments for or against a lifestyle that is compassionate to all creatures is over. We know how to make a difference, to improve our relationship and synergy within the whole. Time to man up!

Do you feel strong and healthy as a vegan man?

I feel strong not only as a man, but as an "earthling". Through my veganism, I have found myself less concerned about appearance and far more concerned about overall balance and well-being. Not only do I feel strong and healthy as a vegan man, my mind is sharper and clearer than ever before.

Are you involved in any work to promote the vegan lifestyle or advance the cause for animals?

Absolutely! I am extremely active both locally and online, with my efforts to promote a better and fairer existence for those we share this place with. Our outreach organization, Vegan by Choice, works on a number of vegan-related initiatives, but advancing the cause for animals is always a top priority and will remain at the top of our list.

Anything else you would like to add?

My evolving practice of veganism has allowed me to find a greater "truth", a truth, that for me, will drive my efforts and quest to restore much of the balance which has become so fractured within our society. I am vegan by choice…it's always choice.

Connect with Josh:

www.veganbychoice.com

The Life-giving Plant-powered Diet is the Natural Choice

David Smugar
USA

Name: David Smugar
Age: 55
Occupation: entrepreneur
Vegan since: 2009 (vegetarian since 2001)
Best thing about being vegan: knowing in my heart that no animal had to suffer or die in order that I may eat. Inspired by a talk given by Howard Lyman.

What are the benefits of being vegan for you?

Knowing that my food choices help reduce methane,

global warming, and water shortages. Water shortages are a worldwide concern. Raising cattle for human consumption is enormously water-intensive. Additionally, I am truly an animal lover, so being vegan just makes good sense.

What is your favourite vegan food?

Vegan "crab" cakes made with garbanzo beans topped with vegan tartar sauce.

What advice would you give men who are considering the switch to the vegan lifestyle?

Just do it. Your manhood will not suffer. On the contrary, you will become more attractive as well as more aware. Oh, and women are intrigued in a good way by a conscientious and sensitive man. Just ask them, and they'll most likely agree.

Do you feel strong and healthy as a vegan man?

Absolutely. I have much more strength and vitality. Animal products consumed many years ago left me feeling sluggish, and milk products created lots of congestion leading to a great loss of energy.

Anything else you would like to add?

Reducing or eliminating meat consumption is crucial to the survival of all beings on our planet. Actress Daryll Hannah was interviewed on a television station called Supreme Master Television regarding her viewpoint on being vegan. She stated that you can't call yourself a true environmentalist unless you follow a vegan diet.

Much of our world's population is not aware, nor sufficiently educated, regarding how detrimental the raising of livestock is on our environment. Heat-trapping gases permeate the atmosphere as a result of the methane produced by animal agriculture.

We pet our dogs, cherish our cats, love our pet birds, bunnies, horses, etc., yet we bake, broil, roast and sauté chickens, ducks, cows, and pigs. Why is that?

The Ethics of Being Vegan

Tim Moore
USA

Name: Tim Moore
Age: 34
Occupation: software developer
Vegan Since: about 16 years
Best thing about being vegan: helping to make the world a more just place for all animals.

What prompted you to make the switch to a plant-powered diet?

I had grown gradually disgusted with the idea of eating meat. When I finally decided to stop eating it for good, a friend of mine that was making the transition from vegetarian to vegan herself gave me a copy of the "Why Vegan?" pamphlet by Vegan Outreach. At first, I thought it might be too much to try to give up all animal-based food at once, but she urged me to try it for a week. I did, and I never looked back. Some other friends were also trying veganism at the same time. It definitely helped to have a supportive group of friends to cook with, go to restaurants with, and share advice. It also helped that students had lobbied the university to have vegan-friendly food in the dining hall.

Do you have any favourite foods?

I love anything made from chickpeas – falafel, hummus, chana masala, or just in a salad. I'm also a big fan of veggie burritos, especially from Papalote in San Francisco or Trippy Taco in Melbourne.

What are the benefits of being vegan for you?

For me it just seems like the obviously right thing to do. There's no moral justification for oppression of animals. Being vegan is the least we can do to start to reverse that wrong.

Do you feel strong and healthy as a vegan man?

I'm no star athlete, but that's been true all my life and has nothing to do with being vegan. I feel very healthy – I rarely get sick and haven't had any physical problems at all. I decided to go vegan for purely ethical reasons, not specifically for my health, but it's had the side-effect of making me more aware and informed about health and nutrition, and that can't be a bad thing!

Are you involved in any work to promote the vegan lifestyle or advance the cause for animals?

I have been on the committee of the Vegan Society

NSW and am a mentor for the Vegan Easy Challenge. I occasionally write about my philosophy of veganism or critique arguments against veganism on my blog at incrementalism.net.

What advice and/or encouragement would you give men that are considering the switch to plant-based living?

It isn't really as hard as you might think, but it definitely helps if you have a friend or two to show you the ropes and give advice. If you don't know anyone personally that can help out, try signing up for the Vegan Easy Challenge at VeganEasy.org. They can set you up with a mentor who you can email with your questions.

Is there anything else you would like to add?

For me, veganism is part of an ethical framework that shapes how I see the world. I like to read books and articles by great vegan thinkers to help me see the practice in its larger context. In my early days as a vegan, I found the writings of Peter Singer really helped to clarify my thinking about the ethical philosophy. If you're interested in understanding more of the ethical basis of veganism, I highly recommend his classic book, *Animal Liberation*. More recently, Melanie Joy has written about "carnism" – the invisible and unchallenged philosophy of meat eaters.

Connect with Tim:

twitter.com/tmoore

"Non-violence leads to the highest ethics, which is the goal of all evolution. Until we stop harming all other living beings, we are still savages."

Thomas Edison

FURTHER READING

Neal D. Barnard. *Dr. Neal Barnard's Program for Reversing Diabetes*. Rodale, 2007.

Ralf Behn. *Unlocking Your Health and Happiness: Holistic Lifestyle for Women and Men's Health*. Mission X Publishing, 2011.

Brendan Brazier. *Thrive: The Vegan Nutrition Guide to Optimal Performance in Sports and Life*. Da Capo Lifelong Books, 2008.

T. Colin Campbell. *The China Study*. Benbella Books, 2006.

Robert Cheeke. *Vegan Bodybuilding & Fitness: The Complete Guide to Building Your Body on a Plant Based Diet*. Healthy Living Publications, 2010.

Harvey Diamond. *Fit for Life*. Kensington (updated edition), 2011.

Caldwell B. Esselstyn, Jr. *Prevent and Reverse Heart Disease*. Avery Trade, 2008.

Rip Esselstyn. *The Engine 2 Diet: The Texas Firefighter's 28-Day Save-Your-Life Plan that Lowers Cholesterol and Burns Away the Pounds.* Grand Central Life & Style, 2009.

Andrew Knight. *The Costs and Benefits of Animal Experiments.* Palgrave Macmillan, 2012.

Howard Lyman. *Mad Cowboy: Plain Truth from the Cattle Rancher Who Won't Eat Meat.* Scribner, 2001.

John Robbins. *Diet for a New America.* H.J Cramer, 1998.

Jeffrey Moussaieff Masson. *The Face on Your Plate: The Truth About Food.* W. W. Norton & Company, Inc., 2009.

Rich Roll. *Finding Ultra: Rejecting Middle Age, Becoming One of the World's Fittest Men, and Discovering Myself.* Crown Archetype, 2012.

Will Tuttle. *The World Peace Diet.* Lantern Books, 2005.

OTHER TITLES BY THE AUTHOR

Forever 21: The empowering guide to reclaiming your youth, beauty, health, happiness and spirituality

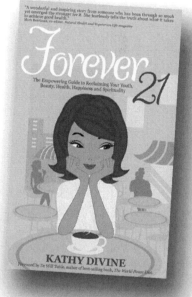

Forever 21 is the book that explains how to look younger, feel happier and healthier while saving animals' lives and helping the environment. The eight Forever 21 Principles give you the tools you need to create a happier and healthier you!

If you are ready to reclaim your power and reach your full potential on every level, this is the book for you!

After being repeatedly told for many years that she looks younger than her age, Kathy Divine decided to document her lifestyle tips for maintaining a youthful look.

Part one of the book elaborates on these secrets of youth, with an explanation of the eight Forever 21 Principles. Part two is a collection of interviews she did with health experts and elite athletes who are focused on empowering people to reach their full potential in all aspects of life.

For more information about *Forever 21* including stockists, see www.kathydivine.com.

***Vegans Are Cool:
A delicious
collection of
essays, interviews
and articles by
cool vegans from
around the planet***

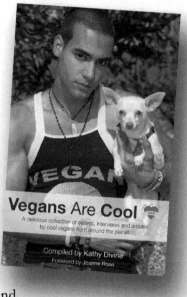

Vegans Are Cool
is a collection of
writings by members
of the global
vegan community.
The aim of this
collaborative project
is to showcase the
knowledge, creativity and
heart of individuals from a diversity of races, cultures
and backgrounds. All the contributors have one thing
in common: they're living the healthy, environmentally
friendly vegan life.

Vegans Are Cool covers the following topics:

* What does being "vegan" actually mean?

* From carnivore to vegan – a how-to guide

* Questions about iron, vitamin B12, protein and vegan
nutrition answered

* Vegan athletes give their top fitness tips

* Weight loss and the vegan diet

…plus much more!

This is *the* vegan how-to guide you can share with your friends and family to show them that going vegan is the way to go! www.vegansarecool.com